Reviews of

The Healing Arts

From birth to death via madness, childbirth, old age, research and nursing, Downie's ambitious scope is matched with powerful poems.

New Scientist

Downie's splendid anthology . . . draws from prose, verse, music, and canvas to link medicine and the arts.

The Lancet

This book is really much better than any anthology has a right to be.

Journal of the Royal College of Physicians of London

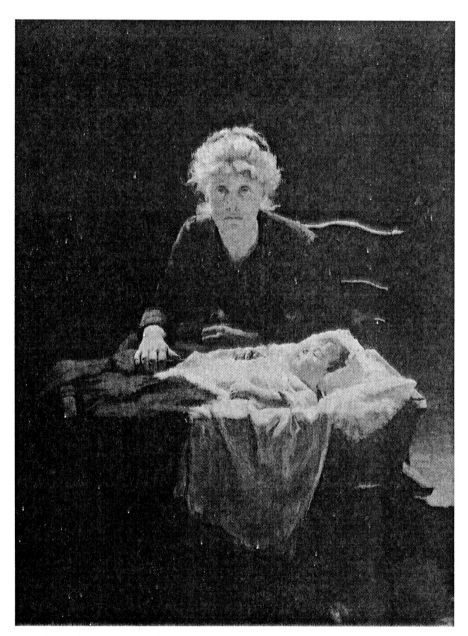

Fantine (1886). *Margaret Bernadine Hall (1863–1910)*

The Healing Arts

An Oxford Illustrated Anthology

Edited by
R. S. DOWNIE

with a
Foreword by
Kenneth C. Calman

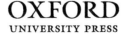

OXFORD
UNIVERSITY PRESS

This book has been printed digitally in order to ensure its continuing availability

OXFORD
UNIVERSITY PRESS

Great Clarendon Street, Oxford OX2 6DP

Oxford University Press is a department of the University of Oxford.
It furthers the University's objective of excellence in research, scholarship,
and education by publishing worldwide in

Oxford New York

Auckland Bangkok Buenos Aires Cape Town Chennai
Dar es Salaam Delhi Hong Kong Istanbul Karachi Kolkata
Kuala Lumpur Madrid Melbourne Mexico City Mumbai Nairobi
São Paulo Shanghai Singapore Taipei Tokyo Toronto

with an associated company in Berlin

Oxford is a registered trade mark of Oxford University Press
in the UK and in certain other countries

Published in the United States
by Oxford University Press Inc., New York

First published 1994
Reprinted (with corrections) 1995
First published as paperback 2000

A catalogue record for this book is available from the British Library

Library of Congress Cataloging in Publication Data
The healing arts: an Oxford illustrated anthology/edited by R. S. Downie.—1st ed.
1. Arts medicine. I. Downie, R. S (Robert Silcock)
R702.5.H43 1994 610—dc20 94-7454

ISBN 0-19-262319-2 (Hbk)
ISBN 0-19-263257-4 (Pbk)

*To my friends in the
Glasgow Literature and Medicine
Group, in gratitude for many
happy hours of discussion*

In the deserts of the heart
Let the healing fountain start

W. H. AUDEN
'*In Memory of W. B. Yeats*'

⊰ FOREWORD ⊱

Kenneth C. Calman

I REALLY love books; their appearance, their feel, their smell, but most of all what's in them. I still get excited when I open a new book. Long ago I discovered that many others felt the same and that in discussing what we'd read, or were about to read, there developed a bond between us. This in itself has given me great pleasure and I have discovered a whole cohort of doctors who might also have enjoyed studying English Literature at University as well as medicine. Around the mid 1980s as a professor in a Faculty of Medicine, I recognized a like mind in the Faculty of Arts, and we decided to embark together on a short course for medical students on Literature and Medicine. Much has come from that course, particularly the friendships which developed. This present book represents one of its most important outcomes.

In setting out our original objectives we recognized that medical students, and of course all other health-care professionals, might benefit from thinking and reading more widely than the narrow confines of a clinical course. Our purpose was to educate in the true sense of the word, 'to bring out' and develop their thinking, in the traditional way of the Scottish University with its emphasis on philosophy and rhetoric. We wished to encourage breadth as well as depth, discussion, debate, and conversation on a broad range of topics. Our students, and we included ourselves in that category, surpassed all our expectations, and we learned a great deal from each other. It was great fun. R. S. Peters in his book *Ethics and Education* makes the point that the measure of the educated person is his or her ability to converse in a civilized and intelligent way on a wide range of subjects. If that was one of the criteria for the course, and this book, then it has succeeded. The illustrations add a further dimension and illuminate the text in a most effective way.

But there is perhaps another function. Doctors, nurses, and other professionals are very busy people, caught up in the lives and the problems of others. They too have lives of their own, and they too need to consider the quality of their own lives.

Literature and the other arts and humanities provide enormous pleasure and relaxation, together with sources of inspiration and creativity.

I hope this book will help to lighten dark hours, give a sense of peace in the middle of a busy life, and assist in fresh thinking and reflection. It will be relevant not only to those with a clinical background, but the general reader will find much of interest between the covers.

It is several years now since I began my own 'Commonplace Book', in which I have recorded comments on what I have read and heard in order to be able to mull them over at leisure. This book, edited by Professor Downie, goes one step further and does much of it for me! In its range of topics, shades of opinion, and moods of sadness and laughter, it will provide a splendid source of pleasure for anyone who is interested in the Healing Arts. I am proud to have been associated with it in some small way.

London, June 1994

⊰ PREFACE ⊱

THE arts can be entertaining, moving, disturbing, consoling, and rich in insight, and the extracts in this anthology have been chosen because each possesses several of these features. But how can the arts be healing? To heal is to make whole, to restore, and that activity is shared by the arts and every kind of health care. Indeed, there is a case for saying that health care is itself an art with a scientific basis.

This anthology, or perhaps 'miscellany' better expresses its variety, will illustrate several types of connection between health care and the arts. For example, some writers or artists have dealt perceptively with disease and illness, and some patients have acquired heightened artistic awareness through the experience of illness. Again, some doctors and nurses have been musicians, artists, or writers, and some writers, artists, or musicians have had medical conditions which have affected their creative work. This anthology will celebrate all these connections and others as well, with the intention of providing a many-faceted entertainment. Although the aim is to give pleasure, I hope through this pleasure to fulfil some serious purposes: to stretch the imagination, deepen the sympathy, and enrich the perceptions of all those, doctors, nurses and others, who care for patients. Perhaps it may also help us all to be more understanding of ourselves. In striving to attain this kind of understanding we are all, doctors, nurses, patients, and the rest of us, striving for the understanding of the artist.

I have confined commentary to brief introductions to each section. It is of the essence of the arts that they speak directly to us, and commentary can be intrusive. Indeed, the extracts have been placed so that they provide a commentary on one another. It has been said that if your only tool is a hammer all your problems become nails. This anthology is intended to illustrate that there can be tools other than scientific ones for dealing with the sickness, anxieties, and tears of human life. The skills for using these tools can be learned from the arts, and the process of learning is both healing and creative of lasting pleasure.

R. S. DOWNIE

EDITOR'S
⊰ ACKNOWLEDGEMENTS ⊱

I SHOULD like first to acknowledge support from the Sir Hugh Fraser Foundation and the Stevenson Citizenship Fund of the University of Glasgow which has made possible Conferences on Medicine and the Arts of which this Anthology is the outcome. Many people have assisted me in the compilation of the Anthology—too many to mention—and I gratefully recognize their help. In particular, I should like to thank Dr Sandra Billington, Dr Kenneth Boyd, Dr Kenneth Calman, Dr Denise Coia and patients, Dr John Dagg, Dr Eileen Downie, Dr Allan Gaw, Dr Johanna Geyer-Kordesch, Dr Brian Hurwitz, Ms Andrea McLaughlin, Dr Jane Macnaughton, Dr Ruth Richardson, Professor Jon Stallworthy, Ms Elizabeth Telfer, Ms Madeleine Young, my departmental secretaries, Anne Southall and Anne Valentine, and the Scottish Poetry Library. The editorial staff of Oxford University Press have been particularly helpful. I hope the Anthology will provide enjoyment and interest commensurate with the effort which all these friends have put into the preparation of the material.

⊰ CONTENTS ⊱

⁓ ILLUSTRATIONS ⁓

⊰ INTRODUCTION ⊱

The most obvious common ground between healing and the arts is morality. Healing in its many forms generates moral problems which the arts can portray through detailed narrative or with dramatic immediacy. It is possible of course to follow the philosophers and think of the resolution of moral questions in terms of the application of principles supported by rational argument. Principles and logic certainly have their place, but the arts can extend our imaginations and deepen our sympathies and these capacities are essential to the wise and humane doctor and the caring nurse. The point here is that philosophers, like biological and social scientists, must stand back from the phenomena and present their accounts in detached prose style. On the other hand, the arts involve us directly and make us vividly and emotionally aware of what it is like to be in the situation which the philosopher and social scientist discuss, of what it means to be ill oneself, or to be a relative or helper of someone who is ill. In this way the arts develop sympathy of the passive or empathetic kind. Now, passive sympathy easily generates motivation to act, and active sympathy, however well meaning, can be blind, clumsy or humiliating unless it is informed by a sensitive understanding of particular situations or relationships. But the arts have this other aspect too: namely, that they can inform sympathy or give it a cognitive shaping. In other words, the arts can develop our perceptions of the complex nature of needs.

Caring for those in need can of course raise questions of the meaning of life, of the tragedy and tears, and sometimes the comic absurdity, built into human relationships. Such questions inevitably arise in medical situations and require some sort of answer if the life of professional care is to seem worthwhile. The arts can approach these questions with an immediacy lacking in the abstractions of philosophy or the social sciences. Moreover, this immediacy can provide a catharsis, a relief from pent-up emotion and tensions, through tears and laughter.

The arts also develop our self-perceptions. The treatment of doctors and nurses by non-medical writers can here be of interest, often salutary interest, to the professions. Doctors are so used to being in positions of power over patients that it is good for them to be made aware that they are also figures of fun. This can encourage a realistic sense of proportion, and many doctors appreciate this. But whereas Chaucer's Doctour of Physik is a portrait tinged with irony, George Eliot's Lydgate is presented as an ideal with which many doctors can still identify—concerned with patients but also pursuing scientific research. He represents the self they still feel to be their true self, despite the cynicism engendered by a life of committee meetings.

Communication is of central importance in health care. This theme runs all through the anthology, for it is one to which the arts can make a major contribution. For example, literature focuses attention on language, on the connotations and resonances of words used to describe or express feelings and fears. Painting, on the other hand, brings out the non-verbal ways in which feelings or attitudes can be expressed. Take, for example, the sympathetic portrayal of the doctor in the painting 'The Doctor' by Sir Luke Fildes, which hangs in the Tate Gallery. As an illustration of the doctor–patient relationship, this has an eloquent sensitivity which communicates itself more directly than a treatise. No amount of science, social science, or medical ethics can succeed in conveying with the subtlety and infinite variety of the arts this basic aspect of human relationships and therefore of doctor–patient relationships.

I have so far been maintaining that the enjoyment of the arts can at the same time enrich the practice of medicine by generating moral questions, by stretching the imagination and deepening the sympathies, by providing a catharsis for the tensions and emotions produced in medical practice, by increasing self-awareness and restoring lost ideals, and by focusing attention on communication. This recapitulation enables me to make explicit the central theme which unifies the whole anthology: it is that medicine is itself an art. Despite the enormous developments in the sciences relevant to medicine (and these are just about all the sciences and social sciences) the simple truth remains: doctors and nurses treat patients and not disease-entities. No matter how well informed in the sciences doctors and nurses are nowadays obliged to become, the actual treatment of patients has the characteristics of art and can be sensitive or insensitive as art can be. This thesis, once upon a time widely recognized in medical education, is now sufficiently contentious to require some further explanation and defence.

First, science by its very essence is concerned with the general, the repeatable elements in nature including human nature; but medicine, using science, is concerned with the particularity, the uniqueness of individual patients. In its concern with the particular and the unique, medicine resembles the arts.

Secondly, in its concentration on the repeatable patterns and laws of nature science must of necessity be impersonal; it records the meaningless processes which would continue whether we were there or not to participate. Medicine, on the other hand, must be concerned with what illness and disease mean for a given patient. This is not to say that disease has a meaning (diseases are impersonal like any other processes which can be understood by science), but it is to say that diseases have meanings for patients. One and the same disease might have quite a different meaning for two patients and therefore different treatments might be appropriate. The arts are vehicles through which human beings articulate the meanings of their lives, and this anthology presents some of the many ways in which disease, illness, birth, and death can be seen.

Thirdly, medicine and the arts are each concerned with healing, with bringing about wholeness. This, the most important point, is made by M. Therese Southgate, a physician and former deputy editor of the *Journal of the American Medical Association*, a medical journal which publishes reproductions of paintings on its cover:

> Medicine and Art have a common goal: to complete what nature cannot bring to a finish ... to reach the ideal ... to heal creation. This is done by paying attention. The physician attends the patient; the artist attends nature. ... If we are attentive in looking, in listening and in waiting, then sooner or later something in the depths of ourselves will respond. Art, like medicine, is not an arrival; it's a search. This is why, perhaps, we call medicine itself an art.

There will of course be objections to what I have claimed for medicine and the arts. I have claimed that the practice of medicine is an art, although an art informed by science. It may be objected that I have at best established only that medicine has some features in common with the arts; perhaps it is better viewed as a craft than an art. Well, this is an introduction to an anthology and not a D.Phil. in philosophy, so I shall be content if the resemblances between the practice of medicine and the arts are noted. They certainly exist in striking parallels if not identities.

I am more concerned with a second objection, that the insight and understanding achieved through the arts is, of all disreputable things, unscientific (and therefore in some sense superficial or spurious). Someone pressing this objection would see the point of the arts as simply giving pleasure 'to them as likes that kind of thing'. Now such an objection does not altogether destroy the justification for this anthology, for I hope it will give pleasure, but it casts doubt on what I have claimed to be its deeper purposes. Enjoyment can have a deep structure; pushpin is not as good as poetry, at least if one wants more than the pleasure of a momentary diversion. Is it true, then, that the insight or understanding achieved through the arts is unscientific?

It is certainly non-scientific because, as I have maintained, scientific understanding is concerned with patterns, with what is repeatable, whereas the kind of understanding which comes from the arts does not arise from what is repeatable but is unique to each situation. But it does not follow from the point that this sort of understanding is non-scientific either that it cannot be based on any evidence or that there is no way of testing it. The evidence will be patients' own accounts of how they see their situations or problems, and testing one's understanding of their situations is a matter of, for example, gauging their reactions to further questions. A knowledge of social science might be a help here, but it is just as likely to be an impediment, because it will encourage the doctor or nurse to see unique individuals and their problems in terms of general categories and labels.

The term 'folk psychology' is sometimes invoked to disparage the kind of insights and understanding which come from the arts. The assumption seems to be that imaginative writers and artists are attempting to do crudely and unsystematically what modern psychologists do in a sophisticated and rigorous manner. This assumption needs only to be stated for its absurdity to be seen. Imaginative writers or artists are not attempting to write systematic treatises on human behaviour, although this does not mean that what they write is not, in another sense, psychology. It is the term 'folk' that is objectionable in the expression, with its suggestion of unlearned naïvety. But the arts abound in refined, accurate, and sensitive analyses of human beings and their relationships and need not be at all simple-minded.

It is important to insist that we can indeed learn from the arts, while denying that they teach us by generalizing from experience. The important question is not 'Can we learn from the arts?' but 'How do we learn from the arts?' The answer to the question thus reformulated is that we learn by imaginative identification with the situations or characters depicted, and by having our imaginations stretched through being made to enter into unfamiliar situations or to see points of view other than our own. Learning of this kind is generative of a deep understanding which is essential to humane nursing and doctoring; it is the key to achieving the 'whole person understanding' which some critics find missing in medical education and medical practice.

⊰ 1 ⊱
The Way We Are

*L*OVE, *birth, youth, and age are not pathological events or processes, but they can be of professional interest to doctors or nurses. Indeed, a large percentage of patients seen by general or family practitioners are within the 'normal' range. Their 'ailments' are the outcomes of the stresses which accompany being alive, and humane advice can be professionally given without 'medicalizing' ordinary problems. The people who speak or are described in this chapter are ordinary people whose experiences and problems are those of all of us, including doctors and nurses. It is appropriate that this is where we begin because this chapter celebrates our ordinary humanity which medicine exists to protect and enhance.*

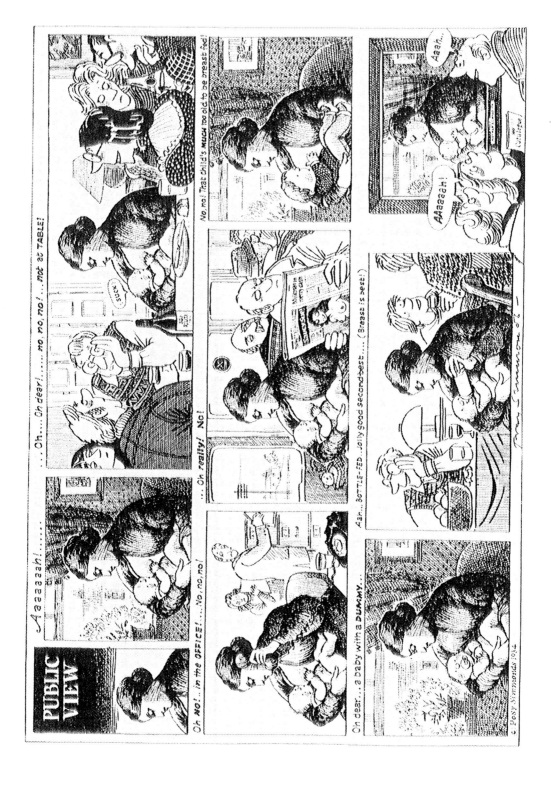

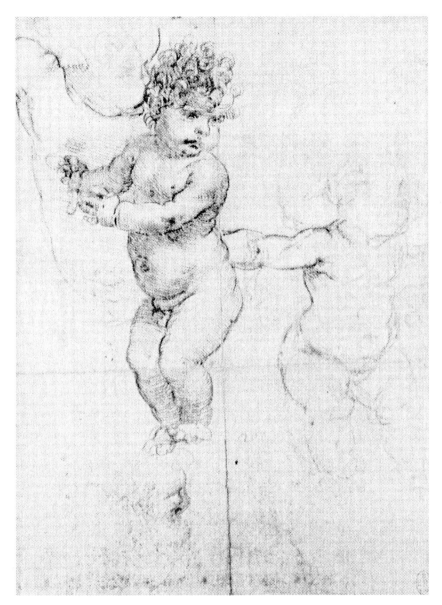

Studies of the Head and Body of a Naked Child (c. 1506–9). *Leonardo da Vinci*
Leonardo noted that the proportions of a baby's body are different from those of an
adult, in that babies are thin at their joints and fat between the joints. He believed that
the proportionately larger head of a baby showed that 'nature first composes in us the
mass of the house of the intellect and then that of the vital spirits'. These studies
are probably preliminaries for the Virgin, Child, and St Anne.

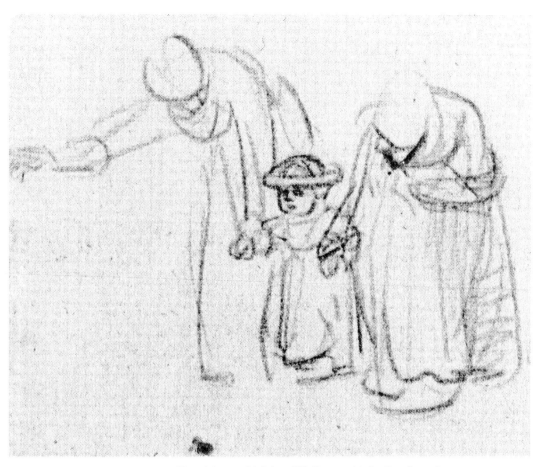

Two Women Teaching a Child to Walk (c. 1637). *Rembrandt*
This drawing displays accurate observation and perfectly conveys a sense of movement.
With very few lines Rembrandt makes us experience the awkwardly stooping movements of the
women and the concentration of the child.

Birth and Childhood

Penelope Shuttle
1947–

First Foetal Movements of My Daughter

Shadow of a fish
The water-echo
Inner florist dancing
Her fathomless ease
Her gauzy thumbs
Leapfrogger,
her olympics in the womb's stadium.

Anne Stevenson
1933–

The Spirit is Too Blunt an Instrument

The spirit is too blunt an instrument
to have made this baby.
Nothing so unskilful as human passions
could have managed the intricate
exacting particulars: the tiny
blind bones with their manipulative tendons,
the knee and the knucklebones, the resilient
fine meshings of ganglia and vertebrae
in the chain of the difficult spine.

Sylvia Plath
1932–1963

Morning Song

LOVE set you going like a fat gold watch.
The midwife slapped your footsoles, and your bald cry
Took its place among the elements.

Our voices echo, magnifying your arrival. New statue.
In a drafty museum, your nakedness
Shadows our safety. We stand round blankly as walls.

I'm no more your mother
Than the cloud that distils a mirror to reflect its own slow
Effacement of the Wind's hand.

All night your moth-breath
Flickers among the flat pink roses. I wake to listen:
A far sea moves in my ear.

One cry, and I stumble from bed, cow-heavy and floral
In my Victorian nightgown.
Your mouth opens clean as a cat's. The window square

Whitens and swallows its dull stars. And now you try
Your handful of notes;
The clear vowels rise like balloons.

Thom Gunn
1929–

Baby Song

FROM the private ease of Mother's womb
I fall into the lighted room.

Why don't they simply put me back
Where it is warm and wet and black?

But one thing follows on another.
Things were different inside Mother.

Padded and jolly I would ride
The perfect comfort of her inside.

They tuck me in a rustling bed
– I lie there, raging, small, and red.

I may sleep soon, I may forget,
But I won't forget that I regret.

A rain of blood poured round her womb,
But all time roars outside this room.

Anne Sexton
1928–1974

The Abortion

SOMEBODY who should have been born
is gone.

Just as the earth puckered its mouth,
each bud puffing out from its knot,
I changed my shoes, and then drove south.

Up past the Blue Mountains, where
Pennsylvania humps on endlessly,
wearing, like a crayoned cat, its green hair,

its roads sunken in like a grey washboard;
where, in truth, the ground cracks evilly,
a dark socket from which the coal has poured,

Somebody who should have been born
is gone.

the grass as bristly and stout as chives,
and me wondering when the ground would break,
and me wondering how anything fragile survives;

up in Pennsylvania, I met a little man,
not Rumpelstiltskin, at all, at all . . .
he took the fullness that love began.

Returning north, even the sky grew thin
like a high window looking nowhere.
The road was as flat as a sheet of tin.

Somebody who should have been born
is gone.

Yes, woman, such logic will lead
to loss without death. Or say what you meant,
you coward . . . this baby that I bleed.

Laurence Sterne
1713–1768

From *Tristram Shandy*

MY father, who dipp'd into all kinds of books, upon looking into *Lithopedus Senonesis de Partu difficili*,* published by *Adrianus Smelvogt*, had found out, that the lax and pliable state of a child's head in parturition, the bones of the cranium having no sutures at that time, was such,—that by force of the woman's efforts, which, in strong labour-pains, was equal, upon an average, to a weight of 470 pounds averdupoise acting perpendicularly upon it,—it so happened that, in 49 instances out of 50, the said head was compressed and moulded into the shape of an oblong conical piece of dough, such as a pastry-cook generally rolls up in order to make a pye of.—Good God! cried my father, what havock and destruction must this make in the infinitely fine and tender texture of the cerebellum!—Or if there is

---

* The author is here twice mistaken;—for *Lithopædus* should be wrote thus, *Lithopædii Senonensis Icon.* The second mistake is, that this *Lithopædus* is not an author, but a drawing of a petrified child. The account of this, published by *Albosius*, 1580, may be seen at the end of *Cordæus*'s works in *Spachius.* Mr. *Tristram Shandy* has been led into this error, either from seeing *Lithopædus*'s name of late in a catalogue of learned writers in Dr. ——, or by mistaking *Lithopædus* for *Trinecavellius*,—from the too great similitude of the names.

such a juice as *Borri* pretends,—is it not enough to make the clearest liquor in the world both feculent and mothery?

But how great was his apprehension, when he further understood, that this force, acting upon the very vertex of the head, not only injured the brain itself or cerebrum,—but that it necessarily squeez'd and propell'd the cerebrum towards the cerebellum, which was the immediate seat of the understanding.—Angels and Ministers of grace defend us! cried my father,—can any soul withstand this shock?—No wonder the intellectual web is so rent and tatter'd as we see it; and that so many of our best heads are no better than a puzzled skein of silk,—all perplexity,—all confusion within side.

But when my father read on, and was let into the secret, that when a child was turn'd topsy-turvy, which was easy for an operator to do, and was extracted by the feet;—that instead of the cerebrum being propell'd towards the cerebellum, the cerebellum, on the contrary, was propell'd simply towards the cerebrum where it could do no manner of hurt:—By heavens! cried he, the world is in a conspiracy to drive out what little wit God has given us,—and the professors of the obstetrick art are listed into the same conspiracy.—What is it to me which end of my son comes foremost into the world, provided all goes right after, and his cerebellum escapes uncrushed?

It is the nature of an hypothesis, when once a man has conceived it, that it assimulates every thing to itself as proper nourishment; and, from the first moment of your begetting it, it generally grows the stronger by every thing you see, hear, read, or understand. This is of great use.

When my father was gone with this about a month, there was scarce a phenomenon of stupidity or of genius, which he could not readily solve by it;—it accounted for the eldest son being the greatest blockhead in the family.—Poor Devil, he would say,—he made way for the capacity of his younger brothers.—It unriddled the observation of drivellers and monstrous heads,—shewing, *a priori*, it could not be otherwise,—unless **** I don't know what. It wonderfully explain'd and accounted for the acumen of the *Asiatick* genius, and that sprightlier turn, and a more penetrating intuition of minds, in warmer climates; not from the loose and common-place solution of a clearer sky, and a more perpetual sunshine, etc.—which, for aught he knew, might as well rarify and dilute the faculties of the soul into nothing, by one extreme,—as they are condensed in colder climates by the other;—but he traced the affair up to its springhead;—shew'd that, in warmer climates, nature had laid a lighter tax upon the fairest parts of the creation;—their pleasures more;—the necessity of their pains less, insomuch that the pressure and resistance upon the vertex was so slight, that the whole organization of the cerebellum was preserved;—nay, he did not believe, in natural births, that so much as a single thread of the network was broke or displaced,—so that the soul might just act as she liked.

When my father had got so far,—what a blaze of light did the accounts of the *Caesarean* section, and of the towering geniuses who had come safe into the world by it, cast upon this hypothesis? Here you see, he would say, there was no injury done to the sensorium;—no pressure of the head against the pelvis;—no propulsion of the cerebrum towards the cerebellum, either by the *oss pubis* on this side, or the *oss coxcygis* on that;—and, pray, what were the happy consequences? Why, Sir, your *Julius Caesar*, who gave the operation a name;—and your *Hermes Trismegistus*, who was born so before ever the operation had a name;—your *Scipio Africanus*; your *Manlius Torquatus*; our *Edward* the sixth,—who, had he lived, would have done the same honour to the hypothesis:—These, and many more, who figur'd high in the annals of fame,—all came *side-way*, Sir, into the world.

This incision of the *abdomen* and *uterus*, ran for six weeks together in my father's head;—he had read, and was satisfied, that wounds in the *epigastrium*, and those in the *matrix*, were not mortal;—so that the belly of the mother might be opened extremely well to give a passage to the child.—He mentioned the thing one afternoon to my mother,—merely as a matter of fact;—but seeing her turn as pale as ashes at the very mention of it, as much as the operation flattered his hopes,—he thought it as well to say no more of it,—contenting himself with admiring—what he thought was to no purpose to propose.

This was my father Mr *Shandy*'s hypothesis; concerning which I have only to add, that my brother *Bobby* did as great honour to it (whatever he did to the family) as any one of the great heroes we spoke of:—For happening not only to be christen'd, as I told you, but to be born too, when my father was at *Epsom*,—being moreover my mother's *first* child,—coming into the world with his head *foremost*,—and turning out afterwards a lad of wonderful slow parts,—my father spelt all these together into his opinion; and as he had failed at one end,—he was determined to try the other.

Pablo Neruda
1904–1973

To the Foot from Its Child

THE child's foot is not yet aware it's a foot,
and would like to be a butterfly or an apple.

But in time, stones and bits of glass,
streets, ladders,
and the paths in the rough earth
go on teaching the foot that it cannot fly,
cannot be a fruit bulging on the branch.
Then, the child's foot
is defeated, falls
in the battle,
is a prisoner
condemned to live in a shoe.

Bit by bit, in that dark,
it grows to know the world in its own way,
out of touch with its fellow, enclosed,
feeling out life like a blind man.

These soft nails
of quartz, bunched together,
grow hard, and change themselves
into opaque substance, hard as horn,
and the tiny, petalled toes of the child
grow bunched and out of trim,
take on the form of eyeless reptiles
with triangular heads, like worms.
Later, they grow calloused
and are covered
with the faint volcanoes of death,
a coarsening hard to accept.

But this blind thing walks
without respite, never stopping
for hour after hour,
the one foot, the other,
now the man's
now the woman's,
up above,
down below,
through fields, mines,
markets and ministries,
backwards,
far afield, inward,
forward,
this foot toils in its shoe,
scarcely taking time
to bare itself in love or sleep;
it walks, they walk,
until the whole man chooses to stop.

And then it descended
underground, unaware,
for there, everything, everything was dark.
It never knew it had ceased to be a foot
or if they were burying it so that it could fly
or so that it could become
an apple.

(Translated from the Spanish by Alistair Reid)

Michel de Montaigne
1533–1592
From *Essays*

I CONDEMN all violence in the education of a tender soul that is being trained for honour and freedom. There is something servile in harshness and constraint; and I believe that what cannot be accomplished by reason, and by wisdom and tact, can never be accomplished by force. That is how I was brought up. They tell me that in all my childhood I was only whipped twice, and then very mildly. I owed the same upbringing to my own children. They all died at nurse, except Leonor, my one daughter who escaped this unhappy fate. She has reached the age of more than 6 without anything but words, and very gentle words, being used to guide her and correct her childish faults. Her mother's indulgence readily concurred in this. And even if my hopes in her should be disappointed, there will be enough other causes for this without blaming my educational system, which I know to be just and natural. I should have followed it still more scrupulously with sons, who are born less subservient and are freer by nature. I should have loved to build up their courage by honest and frank treatment. I have never seen any other effects of a whipping than to make the soul more cowardly and more perversely obstinate.

(Translated from the French by J. M. Cohen)

Fiona Sampson
1963–

Summer House

THE warm house smells of pee
dust and toast. The staircase, old
coiled cat, stretches in heat it's forgotten the feel of.
The house bakes, raises its roof
in the dome of the summer night:
pale toys flower the dark carpet.

When the children climb their magic ladder
into the hair of the house
under the eaves ticking with heat
under the attics filled with the mooing of doves:
they take up the ladder of their imagination
after them.

I climb the stairs
to the edge of my children's secrecy.
They lie unpacked by sleep,
arms loose as mobiles. Their breathing
rustles like small watches.
Above the bunny bag,

between the beds, the window stands open.
Their dreams are streaming out of it,
condensing high in the sky
to rain down
little shops and toys in
intricate uniforms.

Stevie Smith
1902–1971

Advice to Young Children

'CHILDREN who paddle where the ocean bed shelves
   steeply
Must take care they do not,
Paddle too deeply.'

Thus spake the awful aging couple
Whose heart the years had turned to rubble.

But the little children, to save any bother,
Let it in at one ear and out at the other.

Dylan Thomas
1914–1953

Fern Hill

Now as I was young and easy under the apple boughs
About the lilting house and happy as the grass was green,
    The night above the dingle starry,
      Time let me hail and climb
    Golden in the heydays of his eyes,
And honoured among wagons I was prince of the apple towns
And once below a time I lordly had the trees and leaves
      Trail with daisies and barley
    Down the rivers of the windfall light.

And as I was green and carefree, famous among the barns
About the happy yard and singing as the farm was home,
    In the sun that is young once only,
      Time let me play and be
    Golden in the mercy of his means,

And green and golden I was huntsman and herdsman, the calves
Sang to my horn, the foxes on the hills barked clear and cold,
      And the sabbath rang slowly
    In the pebbles of the holy streams.

All the sun long it was running, it was lovely, the hay
Fields high as the house, the tunes from the chimneys, it was air
    And playing, lovely and watery
      And fire green as grass.
    And nightly under the simple stars
As I rode to sleep the owls were bearing the farm away,
All the moon long I heard, blessed among stables, the nightjars
    Flying with the ricks, and the horses
      Flashing into the dark.

And then to awake, and the farm, like a wanderer white
With the dew, come back, the cock on his shoulder: it was all
    Shining, it was Adam and maiden,
      The sky gathered again
    And the sun grew round that very day.
So it must have been after the birth of the simple light
In the first, spinning place, the spellbound horses walking warm
    Out of the whinnying green stable
      On to the fields of praise.

And honoured among foxes and pheasants by the gay house
Under the new made clouds and happy as the heart was long,
    In the sun born over and over,
      I ran my heedless ways,
    My wishes raced through the house high hay
And nothing I cared, at my blue sky trades, that time allows
In all his tuneful turning so few and such morning songs
    Before the children green and golden
      Follow him out of grace,

Nothing I cared, in the lamb white days, that time would take me
Up to the swallow thronged loft by the shadow of my hand,
    In the moon that is always rising,
        Nor that riding to sleep
    I should hear him fly with the high fields
And wake to the farm forever fled from the childless land.
Oh as I was young and easy in the mercy of his means,
      Time held me green and dying
    Though I sang in my chains like the sea.

Philip Larkin
1922–1985

This Be the Verse

THEY fuck you up, your mum and dad.
    They may not mean to, but they do.
They fill you with the faults they had
    And add some extra, just for you.

But they were fucked up in their turn
    By fools in old-style hats and coats,
Who half the time were soppy-stern
    And half at one another's throats.

Man hands on misery to man.
    It deepens like a coastal shelf.
Get out as early as you can,
    And don't have any kids yourself.

Gerard Manley Hopkins
1844–1889

Spring and Fall

to a young child

MÁRGARÉT, áre you gríeving
Over Goldengrove unleaving?
Leáves, líke the things of mán, you
With your fresh thoughts care for, can you?
Áh! ás the héart grows ólder
It will come to such sights colder
By and by, nor spare a sigh
Though worlds of wanwood leafmeal lie;
And yet you will weep and know why.
Now no matter, child, the name:
Sórrow's spríngs áre the sáme.
Nor mouth had, no nor mind, expressed
What héart héard of, ghóst guéssed:
It ís the blíght mán was bórn for,
It is Margaret you mourn for.

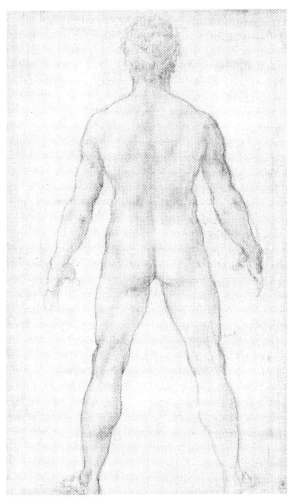

Male Nude Seen from Behind (1503–7). *Leonardo da Vinci*
*This drawing, in red chalk, is an expression of Leonardo's vision of the male body
in full maturity. He and (slightly later) Michelangelo portrayed firmly-muscled
male figures which, apart from their powerful expression of the beauty of the male
body, reveal the widespread interest in anatomy which was shared by sculptors,
painters, and anatomists alike during the High Renaissance. Indeed, some of the
illustrations in Vesalius' famous anatomy textbook* De Humani Corporis Fabrica
*(1543) may have been by Titian and his assistants. Certainly, Vesalius was a
great lover of the arts and the illustrations in his text book are works of art in their
own right.*

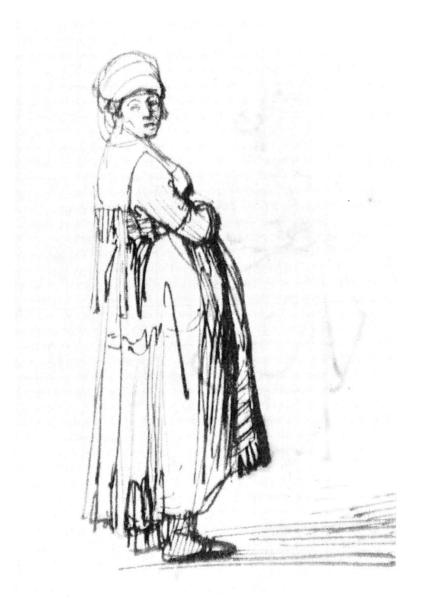

Pregnant Woman Standing (c. 1633). *Rembrandt*
Leonardo's drawings, despite their attention to detail, do not give the impression of drawing as an end in itself. They are the shorthand for his ideas. In contrast, Rembrandt's drawings offer a complete if economical treatment of a subject. These qualities are apparent in A Pregnant Woman Standing.

Love and Marriage

Anonymous
4th Century Chinese

Plucking the Rushes

GREEN rushes with red shoots,
Long leaves bending to the wind—
You and I in the same boat
Plucking rushes at the Five Lakes.
We started at dawn from the orchid-island;
We rested under the elms till noon.
You and I plucking rushes
Had not plucked a handful when night came!

(Translated by Arthur Waley)

Fiona Sampson
1963–

Solent, Evening

BIG boats like officers
in a blue sea. And as if they were irises
a pair of black gulls flap
above the shoreline.

A loveletter should be simple
its sheets open as palms
held up to prove conjuror's
identity. I watch the gold lights make for themselves

pairs in the water's silk.
The boat makes for the jetty.
Love lies like a coin
behind your thumb.

Philip Larkin
1922–1985

Wedding-Wind

THE wind blew all my wedding-day,
And my wedding-night was the night of the high wind;
And a stable door was banging, again and again,
That he must go and shut it, leaving me
Stupid in candlelight, hearing rain,
Seeing my face in the twisted candlestick,
Yet seeing nothing. When he came back
He said the horses were restless, and I was sad
That any man or beast that night should lack
The happiness I had.

                    Now in the day
All's ravelled under the sun by the wind's blowing.
He has gone to look at the floods, and I
Carry a chipped pail to the chicken-run,
Set it down, and stare. All is the wind
Hunting through clouds and forests, thrashing
My apron and the hanging cloths on the line.
Can it be borne, this bodying-forth by wind
Of joy my actions turn on, like a thread
Carrying beads? Shall I be let to sleep

Now this perpetual morning shares my bed?
Can even death dry up
These new delighted lakes, conclude
Our kneeling as cattle by all-generous waters?

Jon Stallworthy
1935–

The Source

'*The dead living in their memories*
are, I am persuaded, the source
of all that we call instinct.'
(W. B. Yeats)

TAKING me into your body
you take me out of my own,
releasing an energy,
a spirit, not mine alone

but theirs locked in my cells.
One generation after
another, the blood rose and fell
that lifts us together.

Such ancient, undiminished
longings—my longing! Such
tenderness, such famished
desires! My fathers in search

of fulfillment storm through
my body, releasing now
loved women locked in you
and hungering to be found.

Robert Graves
1895–1985

A Slice of Wedding Cake

WHY have such scores of lovely, gifted girls
    Married impossible men?
Simple self-sacrifice may be ruled out,
    And missionary endeavour, nine times out of ten.

Repeat 'impossible men': not merely rustic,
    Foul-tempered or depraved
(Dramatic foils chosen to show the world
    How well women behave, and always have behaved).

Impossible men: idle, illiterate,
    Self-pitying, dirty, sly,
For whose appearance even in City parks
    Excuses must be made to casual passers-by.

Has God's supply of tolerable husbands
    Fallen, in fact, so low?
Or do I always over-value woman
    At the expense of man?
                Do I?
                    It might be so.

Anne Stevenson
1933–

The Marriage

THEY will fit, she thinks,
but only if her backbone
cuts exactly into his rib cage,
and only if his knees
dock exactly under her knees
and all four
agree on a common angle.

All would be well
if only
they could face each other.

Even as it is
there are compensations
for having to meet
nose to neck
chest to scapula
groin to rump
when they sleep.

They look, at least,
as if they were going
in the same direction.

Dorothy Parker
1893–1967

Unfortunate Coincidence

BY the time you say you're his,
   Shivering and sighing,
And he vows his passion is
   Infinite, undying—
Lady, make a note of this,
   One of you is lying.

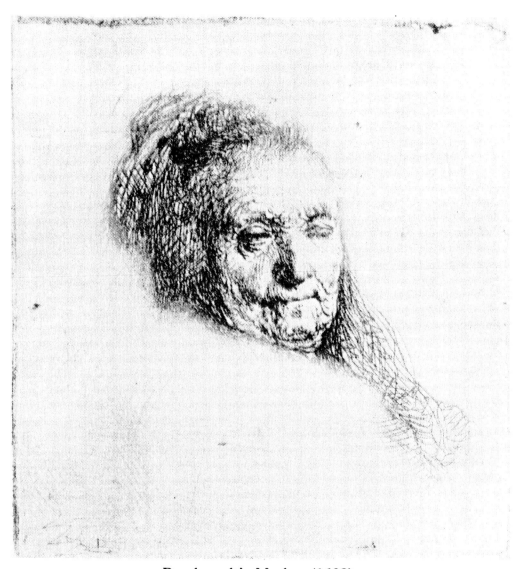

Rembrandt's Mother (1628).
In this etching Rembrandt shows how a needle-drawn line may provide both delicacy and breadth of treatment on small plates. This etching is a realistic but affectionate portrayal of age.

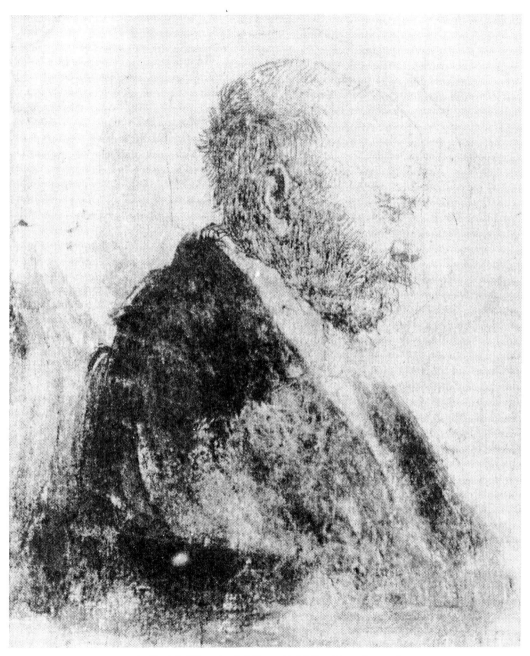

A Bald-Headed Man (1630). *Rembrandt.*
This etching—again a sympathetic portrayal of age—is probably of Rembrandt's father.

Maturity and Age

Philip Larkin
1922–1985

Afternoons

SUMMER is fading:
The leaves fall in ones and twos
From trees bordering
The new recreation ground.
In the hollows of afternoons
Young mothers assemble
At swing and sandpit
Setting free their children.

Behind them, at intervals,
Stand husbands in skilled trades,
An estateful of washing,
And the albums, lettered
Our Wedding, lying
Near the television:
Before them, the wind
Is ruining their courting-places

That are still courting-places
(But the lovers are all in school),
And their children, so intent on
Finding more unripe acorns,

Expect to be taken home.
Their beauty has thickened.
Something is pushing them
To the side of their own lives.

William Shakespeare
1564–1616

Sonnet LXXIII

THAT time of year thou mayst in me behold
When yellow leaves, or none, or few, do hang
Upon those boughs which shake against the cold,
Bare ruin'd choirs, where late the sweet birds sang.
In me thou see'st the twilight of such day
As after sunset fadeth in the west;
Which by and by black night doth take away,
Death's second self, that seals up all in rest.
In me thou see'st the glowing of such fire,
That on the ashes of his youth doth lie,
As the death-bed whereon it must expire
Consum'd with that which it was nourish'd by.
This thou perceiv'st, which makes thy love more strong,
To love that well which thou must leave ere long.

Stevie Smith
1902–1971

Autumn

HE told his life story to Mrs Courtly
Who was a widow. 'Let us get married shortly',
He said. 'I am no longer passionate,
But we can have some conversation before it is too late.'

Edna St Vincent Millay
1892–1950

Sonnet XXIX

PITY me not because the light of day
At close of day no longer walks the sky;
Pity me not for beauties passed away
From field and thicket as the year goes by;
Pity me not the waning of the moon,
Nor that the ebbing tide goes out to sea,
Nor that a man's desire is hushed so soon,
And you no longer look with love on me.
This I have known always: Love is no more
Than the wide blossom which the wind assails,
Than the great tide that treads the shifting shore,
Strewing fresh wreckage gathered in the gales:
Pity me that the heart is slow to learn
What the swift mind beholds at every turn.

Seneca
c.4 BC–AD *65*

From *Letter XII*

WHEREVER I turn I see fresh evidence of my old age. I visited my place just out of
Rome recently and was grumbling about the expense of maintaining the building,
which was in a dilapidated state. My manager told me the trouble wasn't due to any
neglect on his part: he was doing his utmost but the house was old. That house had
taken shape under my own hands; what's to become of me if stones of my own age
are crumbling like that? Losing my temper I seized at the first excuse that
presented itself for venting my irritation on him. 'It's quite clear', I said, 'that
these plane trees are being neglected. There's no foliage on them. Look at those
knotty, dried-up branches and those wretched, flaking trunks. That wouldn't
happen if someone dug round them and watered them.' He swore by my guardian
angel that he was doing his utmost: in everything his care was unremitting but the
poor things were just old. Between you and me, now, I had planted them myself
and seen the first leaf appear on them myself. Then, turning towards the front

door, I said: 'Who's that? Who's that decrepit old person? The door's the proper place for him all right—he looks as if he's on the way out. Where did you get him from? What was the attraction in taking over someone else's dead for burial?' Whereupon the man said, 'Don't you recognize me? I'm Felicio. You used to bring me toy figures. I'm the son of the manager Philositus, your pet playmate.' 'The man's absolutely crazy,' I said. 'Become a little child again, has he, actually calls himself my playmate? Well, the way he's losing his teeth at this very moment, it's perfectly possible.'

So I owe it to this place of mine near town that my old age was made clear to me at every turn. Well, we should cherish old age and enjoy it. It is full of pleasure if you know how to use it. Fruit tastes most delicious just when its season is ending. The charms of youth are at their greatest at the time of its passing. It is the final glass which pleases the inveterate drinker, the one that sets the crowning touch on his intoxication and sends him off into oblivion. Every pleasure defers till its last its greatest delights. The time of life which offers the greatest delight is the age that sees the downward movement—not the steep decline—already begun; and in my opinion even the age that stands on the brink has pleasures of its own—or else the very fact of not experiencing the want of any pleasures take their place. How nice it is to have outworn one's desires and left them behind!

'It's not very pleasant, though,' you may say, 'to have death right before one's eyes.' To this I would say, firstly, that death ought to be right there before the eyes of a young man just as much as an old one—the order in which we each receive our summons is not determined by our precedence in the register—and, secondly, that no one is so very old that it would be quite unnatural for him to hope for one more day . . .

(Translated from the Latin by Robin Campbell)

W. H. Auden
1907–1973

The Model

GENERALLY, reading palms or handwriting or faces
  Is a job of translation, since the kind
    Gentleman often is
  A seducer, the frowning schoolgirl may
    Be dying to be asked to stay;
But the body of this old lady exactly indicates her mind;

Rorschach or Binet could not add to what a fool can see
  From the plain fact that she is alive and well;
    For when one is eighty
  Even a teeny-weeny bit of greed
    Makes one very ill indeed,
And a touch of despair is instantaneously fatal:

Whether the town once drank bubbly out of her shoes or whether
  She was a governess with a good name
    In Church circles, if her
  Husband spoiled her or if she lost her son,
    Is by this time all one.
She survived her true condition; she forgave; she became.

So the painter may please himself; give her an English park,
  Rice-fields in China, or a slum tenement;
    Make the sky light or dark;
  Put green plush behind her or a red brick wall.
    She will compose them all,
Centring the eye on their essential human element.

W. B. Yeats
1865–1939

When You Are Old

WHEN you are old and gray and full of sleep,
And nodding by the fire, take down this book,
And slowly read, and dream of the soft look
Your eyes had once, and of their shadows deep;

How many loved your moments of glad grace,
And loved your beauty with love false or true,

But one man loved the pilgrim soul in you,
And loved the sorrows of your changing face;

And bending down beside the glowing bars,
Murmur, a little sadly, how Love fled
And paced upon the mountains overhead
And hid his face amid a crowd of stars.

Edward Lowbury
1913–

Falls

PULLED by the sky's gravitation
Smoke falls upwards;
The money-spider floats, in perfect balance;
And a child on shaky limbs
Drops into its mother's arms,
Or falls light—no need to fear the fall
When earth is near and motherly.

But no maternal arms
Reach out to save those on shaky limbs
Who fall in second childhood.
The earth is hard and far away beneath them,
The bones are brittle

And every fall brings pain or injury—
Until, at last, light
As smoke, they feel once more
The gravity of the sky
And learn to fall upwards.

Tessa Ransford
1938–

To My Mother, Old and Forgetful
IT'S time to leave and I hug you,
all that is you in my life
as I let it go.

I leave the world as new,
when snowdrops were new and puppies
and travel and books
and my own body was new,
my clothes and shoes
because I was growing.

I leave my sense of home:
your tweeds and brooches,
the paintings you did of trees,
your old desk and three-cornered chair,
the green and white vase for flowers
from the garden you made wherever you lived;

your voice that speaks my name,
your hands, the way they loved
my children and showed it
in deeds over and over.

Before my memory worked
I lived in you, in your mind.
Now I do the remembering

and tell you who you were and
where you are
and what we are doing now,

as I leave you receding
into the future.
It will coil and join up
with the past
and we'll be together
as always.

Jenny Joseph
1932–

Warning

WHEN I am an old woman I shall wear purple
With a red hat which doesn't go, and doesn't suit me.
And I shall spend my pension on brandy and summer gloves
And satin sandals, and say we've no money for butter.
I shall sit down on the pavement when I'm tired
And gobble up samples in shops and press alarm bells
And run my stick along the public railings
And make up for the sobriety of my youth.
I shall go out in my slippers in the rain
And pick flowers in other people's gardens
And learn to spit.

You can wear terrible shirts and grow more fat
And eat three pounds of sausages at a go
Or only bread and pickle for a week
And hoard pens and pencils and beermats and things in boxes.

But now we must have clothes that keep us dry
And pay our rent and not swear in the street
And set a good example for the children.
We must have friends to dinner and read the papers.

But maybe I ought to practise a little now?
So people who know me are not too shocked and surprised
When suddenly I am old, and start to wear purple.

Philip Larkin
1922–1985

At Grass

THE eye can hardly pick them out
From the cold shade they shelter in,
Till wind distresses tail and mane;
Then one crops grass, and moves about
—The other seeming to look on—
And stands anonymous again.

Yet fifteen years ago, perhaps
Two dozen distances sufficed
To fable them: faint afternoons
Of Cups and Stakes and Handicaps,
Whereby their names were artificed
To inlay faded, classic Junes—

Silks at the start: against the sky
Numbers and parasols: outside,
Squadrons of empty cars, and heat,
And littered grass: then the long cry
Hanging unhushed till it subside
To stop-press columns on the street.

Do memories plague their ears like flies?
They shake their heads. Dusk brims the shadows.
Summer by summer all stole away,
The starting-gates, the crowds and cries—
All but the unmolesting meadows.
Almanacked, their names live; they

Have slipped their names, and stand at ease,
Or gallop for what must be joy,
And not a fieldglass sees them home,
Or curious stop-watch prophesies:
Only the groom, and the groom's boy,
With bridles in the evening come.

T. S. Eliot
1888–1965

From *Four Quartets*

[*Little Gidding*]

WE shall not cease from exploration
And the end of all our exploring
Will be to arrive where we started
And know the place for the first time.
Through the unknown, remembered gate
When the last of earth left to discover
Is that which was the beginning;
At the source of the longest river
The voice of the hidden waterfall
And the children in the apple-tree
Not known, because not looked for
But heard, half-heard, in the stillness
Between two waves of the sea.
Quick now, here, now, always—
A condition of complete simplicity
(Costing not less than everything)
And all shall be well and
All manner of thing shall be well
When the tongues of flame are in-folded
Into the crowned knot of fire
And the fire and the rose are one.

⁂2⁂
Disease and Mental Illness

*I*T *is remarkable how little medicine has changed. The classifications, case reports, and general accounts of disease in Hippocrates (fifth century* BC*) and other Greek physicians are all recognizably medicine in the modern sense. Another ancient medical belief is that we can to some extent control our own health by our mode of life. Sometimes this belief can take a dangerous form, as noted by Susan Sontag; illnesses can quite wrongly be seen as expressions of our personalities or even our moral natures. On the other hand, some great creative minds have triumphed despite or even because of their afflictions.*

This is true even of mental illness, which can have many different sorts of cause, but is universally admitted to be a calamity. Social and medical attitudes to the calamity have been well documented, and some are reported in this chapter. There are, of course, no clear dividing lines between mental illness and the obsessions, passions, and mood swings which can affect us all. This chapter contains extracts which express both the tragically pathological and the endearingly eccentric.

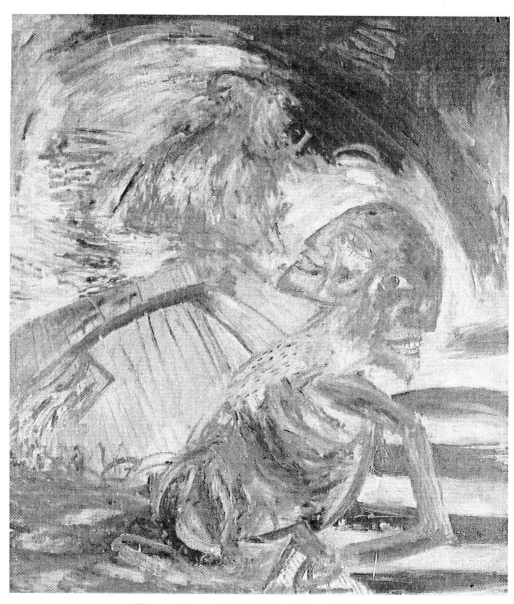

Prometheus II (1988). *John Bellany.*
Prometheus stole fire from Heaven for mankind when they were denied it by Zeus.
Prometheus was punished by being fastened to a rock where an eagle tore daily at
his liver. In 1988 John Bellany, a major British painter, had a highly successful
liver operation carried out in Addenbrooke's Hospital by Sir Roy Calne
(see p. 150).

Disease, Disability, and Plague

Hippocrates
460–357 BC

From *Aphorisms*

THEN, if diseases be grouped according to different age we find that new-born infants suffer from aphthae, vomiting, cough, insomnia, nightmares, inflammation of the umbilicus and discharging ears.

When teething takes place, we must add painful gums, fevers, convulsions, and diarrhoea. These are specially to be expected during the eruption of the canines and in plump children or those with hard bellies.

As they grow older, tonsillitis, deflexions of the vertebrae of the neck, asthma, stone, infection with round worms and ascaris, pedunculated warts, priapism, scrofulous swellings in the cervical glands and other tumours are seen.

On approaching puberty, besides the foregoing diseases we must add long-continued fevers and epistaxis.

Usually children's diseases reach the crisis either in forty days, in seven lunar months or in seven years. Others resolve on the approach of puberty. However, should a disease persist after puberty or, in the case of girls, the time when menstruation is established, it is likely to become chronic.

In youths, haemoptysis, consumption, acute fevers, and epilepsy besides other ailments must be added, but especially those mentioned above.

Later, we encounter asthma, pleurisy, pneumonia, lethargy, inflammation of the brain, *causus*, chronic diarrhoea, cholera, dysentery, enteritis and haemorrhoids.

In the old, dyspnoea, catarrhal coughs, strangury, dysuria, arthritis, nephritis, dizziness, apoplexy, cachexia, pruritus of the whole body, insomnia, ascites and fluid in the eyes and nostrils, failing sight, blindness from glaucoma, and deafness.

(Translated from the Greek by J. Chadwick and W. N. Mann)

Paracelsus
1493–1541
The Nature of Disease

EVEN while still in the womb, man is burdened with the potentialities of every disease, and is subject to them. And because all diseases are inherent in his nature, he could not be born alive and healthy if an inner physician were not hidden in him. But wherever diseases are, there are also physicians and medicine! Each natural disease bears its own remedy within itself. Man has received from nature both the destroyer of health and the preserver of health. And just as the destroyer strives continuously to destroy and to kill man, so the preserver works with equal vigour and zeal to preserve him; what the first strives to shatter and destroy, the innate physician repairs. The destroyer finds in the body the instruments that help him in his destructive work. . . . Just as in the outside world a mason can wreck and has tools for this purpose, just as another mason has tools for building, so both—the destroyer and the preserver—have tools for wrecking and tools for building. . . . The body possesses the high art of wrecking and also of restoring.

   Who can protect himself from harm and disaster if he does not know his enemy? No one. Hence it is indispensable to know him. For there are enemies of many kinds, and it is necessary to know the evil as well as the good. Who can know what joy is, if he has never been sad or in pain? And who can properly discover what God is if he knows nothing of the devil? Just as God reveals to us the enemy of our soul, namely, the devil, so He also reveals to us the enemy of our life, namely, death. And furthermore, He reveals to us the enemy of our body, the enemy of medicine, and the enemy of all natural things. But at the same time He reveals to us by what means this enemy can be disarmed. For there is no sickness against which some remedy has not been created and established, to drive it out and cure it. There is always some remedy, a herb against one disease, a root against another, a water against one, a stone against another, a mineral against one, a poison against another, a metal against one, something else against another.

(Translated from the Latin by N. Guterman)

Bible (Authorized Version)

From *Psalms 22 and 38*

I AM poured out like water, and all my bones are out
  of joint: my heart is like wax; it is melted in the
  midst of my bowels. My strength is dried up like a
  potsherd; and my tongue cleaveth to my jaws . . .

My wounds stink and are corrupt . . . my loins are
  filled with a loathsome disease . . . My heart
  panteth, my strength faileth me; as for the light of
  my eyes, it also is gone from me.

John Milton
1608–1674

On His Blindness

WHEN I consider how my light is spent
  Ere half my days, in this dark world and wide,
  And that one talent which is death to hide
  Lodged with me useless, though my soul more bent
To serve therewith my Maker, and present
  My true account, lest he, returning, chide:
  'Doth God exact day-labour, light denied?'
  I fondly ask: but Patience, to prevent
That murmur, soon replies, 'God doth not need
  Either man's work, or his own gifts; who best
  Bear his mild yoke, they serve him best: his state
Is kingly: thousands at his bidding speed,
  And post o'er land and ocean without rest;
  They also serve who only stand and wait.'

From *Paradise Lost, Bk III*

THUS with the year
Seasons return; but not to me returns
Day, or the sweet approach of even or morn,
Or sight of vernal bloom, or summer's rose,
Or flocks, or herds, or human face divine;
But cloud instead, and ever-during dark
Surrounds me, from the cheerful ways of men
Cut off, and for the book of knowledge fair,
Presented with a universal blank
Of nature's works to me expunged and rased.

Franz Schubert
1797–1828

Letter to Franz von Schober
[*his last letter*]

Vienna, 12 November 1828

Dear Schober,

I am ill. For the last 11 days I have taken nothing to eat or drink; I can only totter feebly from my arm-chair to my bed and back. Rinna is treating me. If I do take any nourishment my body rejects it again at once.

In kindness, let me have some books to ease this desperate situation. Those of Cooper's I have read are *The Last of the Mohicans, The Spy, The Pilot* and *The Settlers*. If by chance you have anything else by him, I do beseech you to leave it for me with Frau v. Bogner at the coffee-house. My brother, who is the soul of conscientiousness, will bring it to me in the most conscientious manner. Or anything else instead.

Your friend
Schubert

(*Translated from the German by Daphne Woodward*)

Ludwig van Beethoven
1770–1827

Letter to Carl Amenda

Vienna, 1 June [1800]

. . . YOUR Beethoven is living most unhappily at odds with Nature and his Creator: several times already I have cursed the latter for exposing His Creatures to the most trifling accidents, whereby the finest flowers are often destroyed and broken. You must know that the noblest part of me, my hearing, has greatly declined; while you were still with me I already had some inkling of this, but said nothing; and now it has grown steadily worse. Whether it is curable remains to be seen; they say it is caused by the condition of my bowels. In that respect I am almost completely cured. As to whether my hearing will now improve as well, I indeed hope so, but faintly: such diseases are the most persistent. How sad my life will be henceforth, deprived of all I love and value, and withal surrounded by such miserable, selfish people. . . . I must say I find Lichnowsky the staunchest of all; since last year he has made me an allowance of 600 fl.; thanks to that and to the ready sale of my work, I need have no anxiety about making both ends meet. Everything I write now I could sell 5 times over at once. . . .

How happy I should now be, if only my hearing were unimpaired. . . . Melancholy resignation, in which I must now take refuge: I have indeed resolved to disregard all this, but how shall I be able to do so? . . . *I beg you to keep the matter of my hearing a great secret and not to confide it to anyone whatsoever.* . . .

(Translated from the German by Daphne Woodward)

Letter to His Friend Dr Franz Wegeler in Bonn

Vienna, 29 June 1800

. . . YOU ask about my circumstances; well, as it happens they are not so bad. Since last year, *Lichnowsky*—who, incredible as you may think it, has always been and still is my warmest friend (there have, indeed, been some slight disagreements between us, but these perhaps only strengthened our friendship)—has made me a guaranteed allowance of 600 fl., on which I can draw until I find a suitable post; my compositions are bringing in a deal of money, and indeed I have almost more commissions than I can satisfy. Moreover, for each work I can have six or seven publishers, or even more if I choose to concern myself with the business; they no longer make agreements with me; I state my terms and they pay up. . . . But now that envious demon, my bad health, has played me a scurvy trick, namely: for the last three years my hearing has grown steadily weaker, and the first cause of this is said to be my bowels, which as you know were already troublesome in the old days, but grew worse after I came here, for I was afflicted with constant diarrhoea which made me extremely weak. . . . Last winter I was in a really poor way . . . until about four weeks ago, when I went to *Vering*. . . . He has almost put a stop to the violent diarrhoea; he ordered me to take warm baths of Danube water, to which I must always add a little bottleful of tonic stuff, gave me no medicine at all until, some four days ago, he prescribed stomach pills and an ear-wash; and, as a result, I certainly feel stronger and better in health—except for my ears, which hum and sing all day and all night. I really lead a wretched life, for nearly two years I have been avoiding almost all company, because I simply cannot tell people I am deaf. If I had any other profession it would be easier, but in my profession this is a terrible situation; and as for my enemies—of whom I have no small number—what would they say about it! . . . If I am at a certain distance from instruments or singers, I cannot hear the high notes; in conversation it is astonishing that there are still people who have never noticed it; I am usually absent-minded, and they put it down to that. Moreover, I can often scarcely hear a person who speaks in a low voice—the tone, yes, but not the words; yet if anyone shouts I find it insupportable. What will happen next, heaven only knows. *Vering says there will certainly be an improvement, if not a complete recovery.* Often already I have cursed my life; Plutarch has taught me resignation. If it proves otherwise I shall brave my fate, though at times I shall be the most unhappy of God's creatures. . . . Resignation! What a miserable refuge, yet it is the only one left for me. . . .

(*Translated from the German by Daphne Woodward*)

Frédéric Chopin
1810–1849

Letter to Albert Cryzmala

Keir, Perthshire, 1 October 1848

. . . I SHALL soon forget all my Polish, I shall be speaking French with an English accent and learn to speak English with a Scots one; in the end I shall be like old Jaworski, who spoke five languages all at the same time. If I do not deluge you with lamentations it is not because you would not try to comfort me: you are the only

person who knows everything about me, but if I once began I should never stop
and it would always be the same thing: for as regards my future, matters are going
from bad to worse. I grow weaker and weaker, and cannot compose anything at all,
not because I do not want to, but owing to practical difficulties: each week I drag
myself to some new perch. What can I do? At least in this way I am saving a few
grosz for the winter. I have received a multitude of invitations, but I cannot even go
where I would like, e.g. to the Duchess of Argyll's or Lady Belhaven's, because it is
already too late in the year for my health. All morning, and until two o'clock, I am
good for nothing, later, when I am dressed, everything oppresses me and I gasp
until dinner, after which I have to sit on at table with the men, watching what they
say and listening as they drink. Sitting there, my thoughts are far away from them,
in spite of all their kindness and their snatches of French: and soon, in the clutches
of a mortal tedium, I go to the drawing-room, where I have to summon all my
moral courage to rouse myself a little, for they are anxious to hear me. Then my
good Daniel carries me up to my bedroom (which is on the floor above, that being
the habit here, as you know), undresses me, puts me to bed, leaves me a candle, and
I am at liberty to gasp and dream until the same thing begins again. No sooner do I
grow a little accustomed to a place than I have to move on, for my Scotswomen
cannot leave me in peace, either they come to fetch me or else they take me on a
round of their families (N.B. where they always get themselves invited too). In the
end they will smother me with their amiability and I, also out of amiability, shall
let them do it. . . .

Letter to His Sister in Warsaw

[Chaillot] Monday 25 June 1849

Mon Âme,

COME, if you can. I feel weak, and no doctor will do me as much good as you. If you
are short of money, borrow some. When I get better I can easily earn some and pay
back whoever lends it to you, but at the moment I am too short to be able to send
you any. My lodgings at Chaillot have room for you, even with two children. . . . I
am sitting in the drawing-room, from where I have a view all over Paris: the
towers, the Tuileries, the Chambre des Députés, St Germain-l'Auxerrois, Saint-
Etienne-du-Mont, Notre-Dame, the Panthéon, Saint-Sulpice, the Val-de-Grâce,
the Invalides, through my five windows; nothing but gardens between us. You will
see when you come. Now attend to the money and the passport, and be quick.

Write me a line at once. . . . God will perhaps let everything go well: if not, behave as though he were doing so. . . .

(*Translated from the French by Daphne Woodward*)

Miroslav Holub
1923–

Vanishing Lung Syndrome

ONCE in a while someone fights for breath.
He stops, getting in everyone's way.
The crowd flows around, muttering
about the flow of crowds,
but he just fights for breath.

Inside there may be growing
a sea monster within a sea monster,
a black, talking bird,
a raven Nevermore that
can't find a bust of Athena
to perch on and so just grows
like the bullous emphysema with cyst development,
fibrous masses and lung hypertension.

Inside there may be growing
a huge muteness of fairy tales,
the wood-block baby that gobbles up everything,
father, mother, flock of sheep,
dead-end road among fields,
screeching wagon and horse,
I've eaten them all and now I'll eat you,
while scintigraphy shows
a disappearance of perfusion, and angiography
shows remnants of arterial branches
without the capillary phase.

Inside there may be growing
an abandoned room,
bare walls, pale squares where pictures hung,
a disconnected phone,
feathers settling on the floor
the encyclopaedists have moved out and
Dostoevsky never found the place,

lost in the landscape
where only surgeons
write poems.

(*Translated from the Czech by David Young and Dana Hábová*)

Susan Sontag
1933–

From *Illness as Metaphor*

THE most striking similarity between the myths of TB and of cancer is that both are, or were, understood as diseases of passion. Fever in TB was a sign of an inward burning: the tubercular is someone 'consumed' by ardor, that ardor leading to the dissolution of the body. The use of metaphors drawn from TB to describe love—the image of 'diseased' love, of a passion that 'consumes'—long antedates the Romantic movement. Starting with the Romantics, the image was inverted, and TB was conceived as a variant of the disease of love. In a heartbreaking letter of November 1, 1820 from Naples, Keats, forever separated from Fanny Brawne, wrote, 'If I had any chance of recovery [from tuberculosis], this passion would kill me.' As a character in *The Magic Mountain* explains: 'Symptoms of disease are nothing but a disguised manifestation of the power of love; and all disease is only love transformed.'

As once TB was thought to come from too much passion, afflicting the reckless and sensual, today many people believe that cancer is a disease of insufficient passion, afflicting those who are sexually repressed, inhibited, unspontaneous, incapable of expressing anger. These seemingly opposite diagnoses are actually not so very different versions of the same view (and deserve, in my opinion, the same amount of credence). For both psychological accounts of a disease stress the insufficiency or the balking of vital energies. As much as TB was celebrated as a disease of passion, it was also regarded as a disease of repression. The high-minded hero of Gide's *The Immoralist* contracts TB (paralleling what Gide perceived to be his own story) because he has repressed his true sexual nature; when Michel accepts Life, he recovers. With this scenario, today Michel would have to get cancer.

As cancer is now imagined to be the wages of repression, so TB was once explained as the ravages of frustration. What is called a liberated sexual life is believed by some people today to stave off cancer, for virtually the same reason that sex was often prescribed to tuberculars as a therapy. In *The Wings of the Dove*, Milly Theale's doctor advises a love affair as a cure for her TB; and it is when she discovers that her duplicitous suitor, Merton Densher, is secretly engaged to her friend Kate Croy that she dies. And in his letter of November 1820, Keats exclaimed: 'My dear Brown, I should have had her when I was in health, and I should have remained well.'

According to the mythology of TB, there is generally some passionate feeling which provokes, which expresses itself in, a bout of TB. But the passions must be thwarted, the hopes blighted. And the passion, although usually love, could be a political or moral passion. At the end of Turgenev's *On the Eve* (1860), Insarov, the young Bulgarian revolutionary-in-exile who is the hero of the novel, realizes that he can't return to Bulgaria. In a hotel in Venice, he sickens with longing and frustration, gets TB, and dies.

Francis Bacon
1561–1626

From *Essays of Deformity*

DEFORMED persons are commonly even with nature: for as nature hath done ill with them, so do they by nature, being for the most part (as the Scripture saith) void of natural affection; and so they have their revenge of nature. Certainly there is a consent between the body and the mind, and where nature erreth in the one, she ventureth in the other: *Ubi peccat in uno, periclitatur in altero.* But because there is in man an election touching the frame of his mind, and a necessity in the frame of his body, the stars of natural inclination are sometimes obscured by the sun of discipline and virtue. Therefore it is good to consider of deformity, not as a sign, which is more deceivable, but as a cause, which seldom faileth of the effect.

Whosoever hath anything fixed in his person that doth induce contempt, hath also a perpetual spur in himself to rescue and deliver himself from scorn. Therefore all deformed persons are extreme bold—first, as in their own defence, as being exposed to scorn, but in process of time, by a general habit. Also, it stirreth in them industry, and especially of this kind, to watch and observe the weakness of others, that they may have somewhat to repay. Again, in their superiors, it quencheth jealousy towards them, as persons that they think they may at pleasure despise; and it layeth their competitors and emulators asleep, as never believing they should be in possibility of advancement, till they see them in possession. So that upon the matter, in a great wit deformity is an advantage to rising. Kings in ancient times (and at this present in some countries) were wont to put great trust in eunuchs, because they that are envious towards all are more obnoxious and officious towards one. But yet their trust towards them hath rather been as to good spials and good whisperers than good magistrates and officers. And much like is the reason of deformed persons. Still the ground is, they will, if they be of spirit, seek to free themselves from scorn, which must be either by virtue or malice. And therefore let it not be marvelled if sometimes they prove excellent persons; as was Agesilaus, Zanger the son of Solyman, Aesop, Gasca, President of Peru; and Socrates may likewise go among them, with others.

William Shakespeare
1564–1616

From *Twelfth Night*, III.

Of Deformity

In nature there's no blemish but the mind;
None can be called deform'd but the unkind:

Susan Sontag
1933–

From *Illness as Metaphor*

According to the mythology of cancer, it is generally a steady repression of feeling that causes the disease. In the earlier, more optimistic form of this fantasy, the repressed feelings were sexual; now, in a notable shift, the repression of violent feelings is imagined to cause cancer. The thwarted passion that killed Insarov was idealism. The passion that people think will give them cancer if they don't discharge it is rage. There are no modern Insarovs. Instead, there are cancerphobes like Norman Mailer, who recently explained that had he not stabbed his wife (and acted out 'a murderous nest of feeling') he would have gotten cancer and 'been dead in a few years himself'. It is the same fantasy that was once attached to TB, but in rather a nastier version.

Jackie Kay
1961–

Dance of the Cherry Blossom
BOTH of us are getting worse
Neither knows who had it first

He thinks I gave it to him
I think he gave it to me

Nights chasing clues where
One memory runs into another like dye.

Both of us are getting worse
I know I'm wasting precious time

But who did he meet between
May 87 and March 89.

I feel his breath on my back
A slow climb into himself then out.

In the morning it all seems different
Neither knows who had it first

We eat breakfast together—newspapers
And silence except for the slow slurp of tea

This companionship is better than anything
He thinks I gave it to him.

By lunchtime we're fighting over some petty thing
He tells me I've lost my sense of humour

I tell him I'm not Glaswegian
You all think death is a joke

It's not funny. I'm dying for fuck's sake
I think he gave it to me.

Just think he says it's every couple's dream
I won't have to wait for you up there

I'll have you night after night—your glorious legs
Your strong hard belly, your kissable cheeks

I cry when he says things like that
My shoulders cave in, my breathing trapped

Do you think you have a corner on dying
You self-pitying wretch, pathetic queen.

He pushes me; we roll on the floor like whirlwind;
When we are done in, our lips find each other

We touch soft as breeze, caress the small parts
Rocking back and forth, his arms become mine

There's nothing outside but the noise of the wind
The cherry blossom's dance through the night.

Robert Burns
1759–1796
Address to the Toothache
Written when the Author Was Grievously
Tormented by that Disorder

My curse upon thy venom'd stang,
That shoots my tortured gums alang;
And through my lugs gies mony a twang,
                    Wi' gnawing vengeance;
Tearing my nerves wi' bitter pang,
                    Like racking engines!

When fevers burn, or ague freezes,
Rheumatics gnaw, or cholic squeezes;
Our neighbour's sympathy may ease us,
                    Wi' pitying moan;
But thee—thou hell o' a' diseases,
                    Aye mocks our groan!

Adown my beard the slavers trickle!
I kick the wee stools o'er the mickel,
As round the fire the giglets keckle,
                    To see me loup;
While, raving mad, I wish a heckle
                    Were in their doup.

Of a' the numerous human dools,
Ill hairsts, daft bargains, cutty-stools,
Or worthy friends raked i' the mools,
                    Sad sight to see!
The tricks o' knaves, or fash o' fools,
                    Thou bear'st the gree.

lugs] ears	loup] jump	ill hairsts] bad harvests
mickle] big	heckle] flax-comb	cutty-stools] stools of repentance
giglets] giggling girls	doup] buttocks	the mools] the grave
keckle) laugh noisily	dools] distresses	to bear the gree] to win the victory

Where'er that place be priests ca' hell,
Whence a' the tones o' misery yell,
And rankèd plagues their numbers tell,
                    In dreadfu' raw,
Thou, Toothache, surely bear'st the bell
                    Amang them a'!

O thou grim mischief-making chiel,
That gars the notes of discord squeel,
Till daft mankind aft dance a reel
                    In gore a shoe thick,
Gie a' the foes o' Scotland's weal
                    A towmond's toothache!

a townmond] a twelve month

Morris Bishop
1893–1944

The Anatomy of Humour

'WHAT is funny?' you ask, my child,
    Crinkling your bright-blue eye.
'Ah, that is a curious question indeed,'
    Musing, I make reply.

'Contusions are funny, not open wounds,
    And automobiles that go
Crash into trees by the highwayside;
    Industrial accidents, no.

'The habit of drink is a hundred per cent,
    But drug addiction is nil.
A nervous breakdown will get no laughs;
    Insanity surely will.

'Humour, aloof from the cigarette,
  Inhabits the droll cigar;
The middle-aged are not very funny;
  The young and the old, they are.

'So the funniest thing in the world should be
  A grandsire, drunk, insane.
Maimed in a motor accident,
  And enduring moderate pain.

'But why do you scream and yell, my child?
  Here comes your mother, my honey,
To comfort you and to lecture me
  For trying, she'll say, to be funny.'

The Plague of 1665

Samuel Pepys
1633–1703

From *Diary*

12 August 1665. THE people die so, that now it seems they are fain to carry the dead to be buried by daylight, the nights not sufficing to do it in. And my Lord Mayor commands people to be within at 9 at night, all (as they say) that the sick may have liberty to go abroad for ayre.

15 August. Up by 4 a'clock and walked to Greenwich, where called at Captain Cockes and to his chamber, he being in bed—where something put my last night's dream into my head, which I think is the best that ever was dreamed—which was, that I had my Lady Castlemayne in my armes and was admitted to use all the dalliance I desired with her, and then dreamed that this could not be awake but that it was only a dream. But that since it was a dream and that I took so much real pleasure in it, what a happy thing it would be, if when we are in our graves (as Shakespeere resembles it), we could dream, and dream but such dreams as this— that then we should not need to be so fearful of death as we are this plague-time.

16 August. Up; and after doing some necessary business about my accounts at home, to the office and there with Mr Hater wrote letters. And I did deliver to him my last will, one part of it to deliver to my wife when I am dead. Thence to the Exchange, which I have not been a great while. But Lord, how sad a sight it is to see the streets empty of people, and very few upon the Change—jealous of every door that one sees shut up, lest it should be the plague—and about us, two shops in three, if not more, generally shut up.

3 September. Lords Day. Up, and put on my coloured silk suit, very fine, and my new periwigg, bought a good while since, but darst not wear it because the plague was in Westminster when I bought it. And it is a wonder what will be the fashion after the plague is done as to periwigs, for nobody will dare to buy any haire for fear of the infection—that it had been cut off of the heads of people dead of the plague. Church being done, my Lord Brouncker, Sir J. Mennes, and I up to the vestry at the desire of the Justices of the Peace, Sir Th. Bidolph and Sir W. Boreman and Alderman Hooker—in order to the doing something for the keeping of the plague from growing; but Lord, to consider the madness of people of the town, who will (because they are forbid) come in crowds along with the dead corps to see them buried. But we agreed on some orders for the prevention thereof.

16 October. But Lord, how empty the [city] streets are, and melancholy, so many poor sick people in the streets, full of sores, and so many sad stories overheard as I walk, everybody talking of this dead, and that man sick, and so many in this place, and so many in that. And they tell me that in Westminster there is never a physitian, and but one apothecary left, all being dead—but that there are great hopes of a great decrease this week: God send it.

5 November. Lords Day. Up, and after being trimmed, by boate to the Cockepitt, where I heard the Duke of Albemarle's chaplain make a simple sermon. Among other things, reproaching the imperfection of humane learning, he cried—'All our physicians can't tell what an ague is, and all our arithmetique is not able to number the days of a man'—which, God knows, is not the fault of arithmetique, but that our understandings reach not that thing. To dinner, where a great deal of silly discourse. But the worst is, I hear that the plague encreases much at Lambeth, St Martins, and Westminster, and fear it will all over the City. Thence I to the Swan, there thinking to have seen Sarah, but she was at church; and so by water to Deptford, and there made a visit to Mr Evelings, who, among other things, showed me most excellent painting in little, in distemper, Indian incke, water colours, graveing; and above all, the whole secret of mezzotinto and the manner of it, which is very pretty, and good things done with it. He read me part of a play or two of his making, very good, but not as he conceits them I think, to be. He showed me his *Hortus Hyemalis*; leaves laid up in a book of several plants, kept dry, which preserve colour however, and look very finely, better than any herbal. In fine, a most excellent person he is, and must be allowed a little for a little conceitedness; but he may well be so, being a man so much above others. He read me, though with too much gusto, some little poems of his own, that were not transcendent, yet one or two very pretty epigrams. Here comes in in the middle of our discourse, Captain Cocke, as drunk as a dog, but could stand and talk and laugh. He did so joy himself in a brave woman that he had been with all the afternoon, and who should it be but my Lady Robinson. But very troublesome he is with his noise and talk and laughing, though very pleasant. With him in his coach to Mr Glanvills, where he sat with Mrs Penington and myself a good while, talking of this fine woman again, and then went away. Then the lady and I to very serious discourse; and among other things, of what a bonny lass my Lady Robinson is, who is reported to be kind to the prisoners, and hath said to Sir G. Smith, who is her great chrony: 'Look, there is a pretty man; I could be contented to break a commandment with him'— and such loose expressions she will have often. After a hour's talk, we to bed—the lady mightily troubled about a little pretty bitch she hath, which is very sick and will eat nothing. And the jest was, I could hear her in her chamber bemoaning the bitch; and by and by taking her to bed with her, the bitch pissed and shit abed, and she was fain to rise and had coals out of my chamber to dry the bed again.

5 January 1666. I, with my Lord Brouncker and Mrs Williams, by coach with four horses to London, to my Lord's house in Covent Garden. But Lord, what staring to see a nobleman's coach come to town—and porters everywhere bow to us, and such begging of beggars. And a delightful thing it is to see the town full of people again, as now it is, and shops begin to open, though in many places, seven or eight together, and more, all shut; but yet the town is full compared with what it used to be—I mean the City end, for Covent Gu[a]rden and Westminster are yet very empty of people, no Court nor gentry being there.

22 January. To the Crowne tavern behind the Exchange by appointment, and there met the first meeting of Gresham College since the Plague. Dr Goddard did fill us with talk in defence of his and his fellow physicians' going out of town in the plague-time; saying that their perticular patients were most gone out of town, and they left at liberty—and a great deal more, etc. But what, among other fine discourse, please me most, was Sir G. Ent about respiration; that it is not to this day known or concluded on among physicians, nor to be done either, how that action is managed by nature or for what use it is. Here late, till poor Dr Merritt was drunk; and so all home and I to bed.

23 January. Up, and to the office and then to dinner. After dinner, to the office again all the afternoon, and much business with me. Good news, beyond all expectation, of the decrease of the plague; being now but 79. So home with comfort to bed. A most furious storme all night and morning.

A Case Study : Beethoven

Dr John Dagg
1933–

Introduction

To many, Beethoven is quite simply the greatest composer in history, dwarfing the attainments of his predecessors and his successors alike. Even if he were not accorded this unique position, his musical persona is indeed Titanic, bridging, as he did, the fading Classical age and the flowering Romantic one, and effecting a revolution in music as profound as the French Revolution had in politics. Above all, his works achieve a supreme nobility and vision which appeal universally to all with ears to hear. That this was achieved from a human frame of such frailty is a matter for wonder, and it is in this spirit that the following note on his medical history is presented.

BEETHOVEN: THE MAN

The personality of Beethoven was vastly complex, with a mass of contradictory and conflicting elements. He suffered wide mood swings from elation to deep despondency during which he became unable to compose, and in twentieth-century jargon would probably be regarded as manic-depressive. Headstrong and impulsive, suspicious and hostile, he was at the same time hypersensitive and easily wounded. Often generous in impulse, yet violent in temper, he was isolated by his genius, his pride, and of course his humiliating deafness. As he himself ruefully remarked he was 'bad at everything except music'.

Dapper in his youth and renowned in society as a pianist, his deafness drove him from the public world of performance into the private one of musical imagination and composition, and into increasing financial and domestic muddle. He could not keep servants, and a home visit in the later part of his life would have revealed considerable chaos; several contemporary accounts describe plates of half-eaten food about the house, an unemptied chamber pot under the piano, spilled water on the floor from his habit of dousing his head in a bowl, and broken strings curling from the piano 'like a thornbush torn in the wind' damaged by his attempts to hear his own playing. Overall he was not penniless and he was helped by kind patrons, who often braved rebuffs to support him; however, financial confusion and the costs of a prolonged lawsuit to wrest custody of his nephew Karl from his widowed sister-in-law did lead to chronic difficulties with money.

RELATIONSHIPS WITH HIS DOCTORS

Over his life time, he had predictably uneasy relationships with at least fifteen doctors; having been insulted, many refused to visit him again. Three names are important—Dr Malfatti, Dr Wegeler, and Dr Wawruch. The first, Dr Giovanni Malfatti (1775–1859), was a fashionable Italian society physician who met Beethoven through a mutual friend; Therese, Malfatti's young niece, was the object of Beethoven's affections and the probable dedicatee of the piano piece 'Für Elise'. In 1810 came the inevitable quarrel—'I changed my doctor, because mine, a wily Italian, had powerful secondary motives, and lacked both honesty and intelligence'. Like Beethoven himself, Dr Franz Wegeler (1765–1848) came from Bonn and was a childhood friend; he later married the sister of Beethoven's friend, Stephan von Breuning. Dr Andreas Wawruch (?–1842), an obese amateur cellist, was summoned to Beethoven's last illness by his nephew Karl, and was heartily loathed by Beethoven; he did, however, write a useful account of Beethoven's terminal illness, in a somewhat pompous and overblown style.

SOURCES OF MEDICAL INFORMATION

There was never any doubt during his lifetime that Beethoven was a great man, and there is much contemporary writing about him, including some information about his illnesses. Secondly, there are the famous conversation books, used by Beethoven's visitors to conduct a dialogue with the deaf composer; obviously these do not contain Beethoven's contributions, but much can be inferred even from one-sided entries. Around half of the four hundred conversation books were destroyed after Beethoven's death by his amanuensis Schindler, presumably in a mistaken attempt to remove any record of compromising or indeed seditious material. Lastly, we have Beethoven's own writings and letters which allude not infrequently to his sufferings.

Case Report

The references to Beethoven's health are scattered over many years but can be drawn together into three main groups.

ABDOMINAL SYMPTOMS

Beethoven first developed abdominal colic and diarrhoea at the age of 21, and ten years later there are further allusions to colic, violent diarrhoea, and severe prostration. In a letter to Dr Wegeler in 1801 Beethoven describes his symptoms and incidentally gives some views on the medical treatment of the time.

> Only that jealous demon, namely my bad health, has thrown a mean spoke in the wheel; in the past three years my hearing has become increasingly weaker. It appears that the abdomen, which, as you know, was already in a wretched state, has become worse here. I have been constantly plagued by colic and hence by a fearful fatigue. Frank wanted to build up the tone of my body by means of strong tonic medicines, and my hearing with almond oil. But Prosit! it did me no good whatever. My hearing became even worse and the digestive trouble remained the same. This went on all last year until the autumn when sometimes I was reduced to utter despair. Then a medical asinus recommended cold baths for my condition; a more intelligent one suggested the usual tepid Danube baths. These worked wonders. I improved, but my deafness persisted or even worsened. This winter I was really wretched. I had fearful colics and I again relapsed completely into my former state. This went on until about four weeks ago, when I went to Vering, since I began to think that this condition might call for a surgeon and, anyway, I always had confidence in him. He succeeded in almost checking the violent diarrhoea. He prescribed the tepid Danube baths into which I must pour a flask of strengthening substances. He gave me no medicines until about four days ago when he prescribed four pills daily for the stomach and an infusion for my ear. I must say that now I find myself stronger and better. Only my ears hum and buzz continuously day and night.

Three years later, when Beethoven was 31, there are further references to fever and the first mention of liver malfunction. This is contained in a letter from Beethoven's friend Stephan von Breuning to Dr Wegeler. 'He (Beethoven) had hardly been with me when he came down with a very serious passing illness, bordering on the fatal, which finally turned into a continuous intermittent fever (his chronic tendency to liver malfunction from old times is noticeable). Worry and nursing rather took it out of me. Now he is quite well again'. NB: The sentence in parentheses was added by Stephan's son, Dr Gerhard von Breuning.

Between 1815 and 1820, he had recurrent musculo-skeletal pains and fever, and in 1821 was again severely ill with jaundice. In 1823 he developed painful eyes and photophobia, occasioning a visit to take the waters at Baden.

By 1825 his health was beginning to deteriorate more seriously; there is a mention of haemoptysis and epistaxis, and in a letter from Beethoven to his nephew Karl, of marked weight loss. At this time he was seen by Professor Braunhofer, Physician and Professor of Biology, and there is an illuminating entry from the Professor in the conversation books; Beethoven is advised to take no wine or coffee, to stick to his diet, and is told he has a 'severe inflammation of the bowels'. His condition continued to undergo remissions as well as relapses, however; in the autograph copy of the late String Quartet in A minor Op 132, over the slow movement Beethoven has inscribed the words 'Song of thanksgiving offered by a convalescent to the Divinity, in the Lydian mode'. Clearly he felt reprieved from death.

The year 1826–7 was to prove the last in Beethoven's life. Following a suicide attempt by his beloved nephew Karl, Beethoven travelled in a farm cart from Gneixendorf to Vienna and became chilled. Thereafter followed continually deteriorating health, and he developed gross abdominal swelling, jaundice, continuing diarrhoea, 'pleurisy', and marked leg swelling. Dr Wawruch's questions to Beethoven (although in Karl's writing) are illuminating.

DIE FÜSSE WAREN NICHT GESCHWOLLEN?
—Have your feet been swelling?
SEIT WANN DER BAUCH SO GESPANNT?
—How long has your belly been so swollen?

The help of Seibert, a general surgeon, was sought, and the abdomen was tapped four times with the removal of around twenty-five pounds (twelve litres) on each occasion. This must have caused great discomfort because fluid leaked continuously into the bed on each occasion and the wound became gangrenous. Beethoven, however, was able to say that it reminded him of 'Moses striking the rock with his staff to bring forth water'. At around this time, Dr Malfatti was persuaded to return and, in the best medical tradition, discontinued his predecessor's therapy, and prescribed sauna baths and iced punch, a humane touch. It is important to note that coma did not supervene until late. Even during the final stages of the illness, Beethoven continued to plan a tenth symphony and was capable of writing a will a few days before his death. This will clearly shows the hand of a troubled man, with the writing trailing off at the right of the page, but there is no tremor or other abnormality to suggest hepatic neuro-encephalopathy. Finally, however, he lost consciousness on 24 March 1827 and died in the presence of his mourning friends two days later.

We can return to Dr Wawruch for two other clinical observations—'At the morning visit I found him in great distress. . . . Shivering and trembling, he writhed with pains which raged in the liver and the bowels, and his hitherto only moderately bloated feet were massively swollen.' 'From this point on developed the dropsy, urinary output became diminished, the liver presented distinctly signs of hard knots, the jaundice increased.' In other words, knobs on the liver were palpable through the abdominal wall.

DEAFNESS

At the age of 27 Beethoven began to note hearing loss; this was only slowly progressive, and initially at least selective for high-pitched sounds. This was accompanied by tinnitus, which he found even more intolerable. His despair is well illustrated by a will written at the village of Heiligenstadt in 1802, known subsequently as the Heiligenstadt Testament.

> My heart and soul, since my childhood, have ever been filled with tender feelings of goodwill; I was ever ready to perform great deeds. But consider that for six years now I have been afflicted with an incurable condition, made worse by incompetent physicians, deceived for year after year by the hope of an improvement and now obliged to face the prospect of permanent disability. Born with an ardent and lively temperament and also inclined to the distractions of society, I am at an early age obliged to seclude myself and live my life in solitude. If once in a while I attempted to ignore all this, Oh how harshly would I be driven back by the doubly sad experience of my bad hearing; yet it was not possible for me to say Speak louder, Shout, because I am deaf. Alas, how would it be possible for me to admit to a weakness of the one sense that should be perfect to a higher degree in me than in others, the one sense which I once possessed in the highest perfection, a perfection that few others of my profession have ever possessed. No I cannot do it. So forgive me if you see me draw back from your company which I would so gladly share. My misfortune is doubly hard to bear, inasmuch as I will surely be misunderstood. For me there can be no recreation in the society of others, no intelligent conversation, no mutual exchange of ideas; only as much as is required by the most pressing needs can I venture into society. I am obliged to live like an outcast. If I venture into the company of men, I am overcome by a burning terror, inasmuch as I fear to find myself in the danger of allowing my condition to be noticed. So it has been for this half year which I have spent in the country. I am advised by my sensible physician

to spare my hearing as much as possible, he to a certain extent encouraged my natural disposition; sometimes torn by the desire for companionship, I allowed myself to be tempted into it. But what a humiliation when someone standing next to me could hear from a distance the sound of a flute, whereas I heard nothing. Or, someone could hear the shepherd singing and that also I did not hear. Such experiences brought me near to despair. It would have needed little for me to put an end to my life.

By 1810 public participation in music making had become impossible, and there are several heart-rending contemporary accounts of disastrous performances as conductor or pianist. By 1822 he was profoundly deaf, although his speech remained normal and he continued to make use of an ear trumpet. The symptoms are compatible with otosclerosis.

SKIN

Early portraits show no skin abnormality but this could have been to flatter the sitter. Later in life, his face was scarred and highly coloured, with the 'terrifying countenance of a leper'. It was common at the time to attribute such appearances to smallpox. His features became coarser as he aged, and the death mask clearly shows atrophic discrete and confluent scars, as well as tissue thickening around the nose and lower face.

Post-Mortem Examination

This was carried out by Dr Johann Wagner, and the subsequently more famous Dr Rokitansky, of the University of Vienna. Despite the paracenteses, there were four quarts of turbid fluid remaining in the abdomen. The gut was dilated and gas filled. The liver was shrunken to half size, but 'beset with knots, the size of a bean'. The spleen was double normal size, and the gall-bladder filled with gravelly sediment. The pancreas was indurated. In modern terminology, death was thus due to macronodular hepatic cirrhosis associated with splenomegaly, probably due to portal hypertension. Marked oedema and ascites were present, and the end was no doubt hastened by peritoneal infection and depletion of fluid and electrolyte occasioned by massive abdominal paracenteses. The gut was dilated, probably secondary to ileus.

The auditory nerves were reported as atrophied and shrivelled on the original report. Extraordinarily, the grave was reopened in 1863 and again in 1888; the skull was in several pieces but on neither occasion could the temporal bones be discovered.

INTERPRETATION

If a single diagnosis can be attempted, it has to take account of an episodic prostrating diarrhoeal illness, recurring jaundice over several years, various less severe symptoms in other areas, and death from macronodular cirrhosis with liver failure. In the opinion of the present writer, chronic ulcerative colitis with one of the cirrhoses associated with it, e.g. sclerosing cholangitis or chronic active hepatitis would fit the picture most closely. Other forms of auto-immune multi-system disorder are possible, but would not take account of the very prominent bowel symptoms. The family history of alcoholism, the irascibility, red face, and domestic and personal disorder could point to alcohol abuse, but the type of cirrhosis is wrong, and the continued function at a superlative intellectual level throughout most of his life makes this very unlikely; Beethoven did drink wine and wine merchants' bills were discovered in his quarters after his death, but there are no contemporary indications that he was habitually intoxicated. Finally syphilis, both congenital and acquired, has been adduced as an explanation for his systemic symptoms and his deafness, and this is the hardest possibility to refute; one wonders if the conversation books destroyed by Schindler might have cast light on this possibility. Space does not permit a full evaluation of the claims of syphilis, but in general it provides a poor explanation of the chronology and behaviour of the clinical picture.

Postlude

The funeral service was held on 29 March 1827 in Vienna. It was attended by an estimated 40,000 mourners and an ovation was given by the Austrian poet Grillparzer—a striking contrast with the shoddy obsequies and unmarked pauper's grave accorded to Mozart. The funeral invitation circulated by 'L van Beethoven's worshippers and friends' concluded as follows: 'The irretrievable loss to the world of the celebrated tone-master took place on the 28th March 1827 at 6 pm. Beethoven died in consequence of dropsy in the fifty-sixth year of his life after having received the Holy Sacrament.'

For much of his creative life, Beethoven was on the rack, physically and emotionally; he was even deprived of the comfort of hearing his own music. His Olympian musical energy, imagination and innovation triumphed over it all to our infinite enrichment and pleasure.

[John H. Dagg is Consultant Physician at the Western Infirmary, Glasgow.]

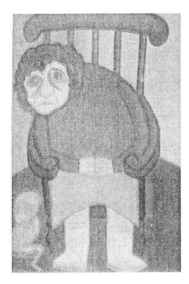
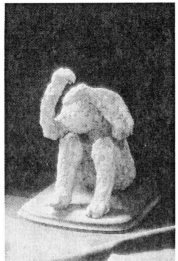
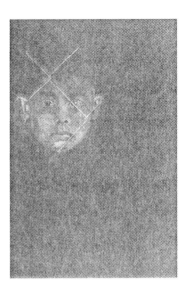

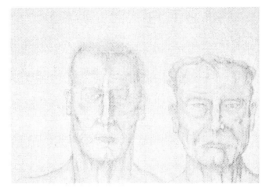

(*Top left.*) Depression. *Anonymous.*
This represents the feelings of her return to the womb.

(*Top centre.*) Leave Me Alone. *Alan Freestone and Alyson.*
This is a photograph of a papier mâché sculpture on depression by an artist working at Edinburgh Royal Infirmary.

(*Top right.*) The Other Side of the Fence. *Stuart C. Jebbitt.*
The artist was a student at Chelsea College of Art. He was brought up in a house where his father was said to be 'mad', and he always felt that there was a barrier there and that he didn't understand what was going on. This painting was bought by a criminal lawyer!

(*Bottom.*) Waiting for ECT. *Stuart Glasgow.*
This is a self-explanatory painting by a patient.

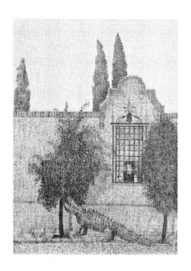

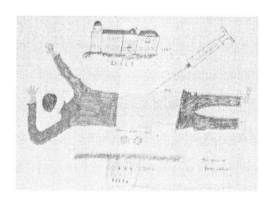

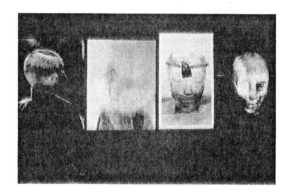

(*Left.*) Girl Looking out of a Window. *Annie Rae.*
This is one of a series of paintings set in Alhambra. The alligator in each of the paintings was a recurrent image in her dreams. The patient, who was a professional artist, was severely depressed and painted only in black and white. The oranges in this painting represent a major step towards the healing of her mind after many years.

(*Top right.*) The Fall of Peter Martin. *Peter Martin.*
This is a complex painting by a patient. Most obviously it brings out the overwhelming impotence of the patient and the indignity of having things done to you. But on the other hand it is the injection which comes between the mental hospital in the background of the picture and the gutter which is in the foreground.

(*Bottom right.*) Chained by Schizophrenia.
This is one of a series of photographs by a relative of a schizophrenic.

The Sick Mind

Adam Smith
1723–1790

The Loss of Reason

OF all the calamities to which the condition of mortality exposes mankind, the loss of reason appears, to those who have the least spark of humanity, by far the most dreadful; and they behold that last stage of human wretchedness with deeper commiseration than any other. But the poor wretch, who is in it, laughs and sings, perhaps, and is altogether insensible to his own misery. The anguish which humanity feels, therefore, at the sight of such an object, cannot be the reflection of any sentiment of the sufferer. The compassion of the spectator must rise altogether from the consideration of what he himself would feel if he was reduced to the same unhappy situation, and, what perhaps is impossible, was at the same time able to regard it with his present reasoned judgement.

(From *The Theory of Moral Sentiments*, 1790)

Theodore Roethke
1908–1963

In a Dark Time

IN a dark time, the eye begins to see,
I meet my shadow in the deepening shade;
I hear my echo in the echoing wood—
A lord of nature weeping to a tree.
I live between the heron and the wren,
Beasts of the hill and serpents of the den.

What's madness but nobility of soul
At odds with circumstance? The day's on fire!
I know the purity of pure despair,
My shadow pinned against a sweating wall.
That place among the rocks—is it a cave,
Or winding path? The edge is what I have.

A steady storm of correspondences!
A night flowing with birds, a ragged moon,
And in broad day the midnight come again!
A man goes far to find out what he is—
Death of the self in a long, tearless night,
All natural shapes blazing unnatural light.

Dark, dark my light, and darker my desire.
My soul, like some heat-maddened summer fly,
Keeps buzzing at the sill. Which I is *I*?
A fallen man, I climb out of my fear.
The mind enters itself, and God the mind,
And one is One, free in the tearing wind.

Oliver Sacks
1933–

From *The Man Who Mistook His Wife for a Hat*

'CAN I help?' I asked.

'Help what? Help whom?'

'Help you put on your shoe.'

'Ach,' he said, 'I had forgotten the shoe', adding, *sotto voce*, 'The shoe? The shoe?' He seemed baffled.

'Your shoe,' I repeated. 'Perhaps you'd put it on.'

He continued to look downwards, though not at the shoe, with an intense but misplaced concentration. Finally his gaze settled on his foot: 'That is my shoe, yes?'

Did I mis-hear? Did he mis-see?

'My eyes,' he explained, and put a hand to his foot, '*This* is my shoe, no?'

'No, it is not. That is your foot. *There* is your shoe.'

'Ah! I thought that was my foot.'

Was he joking? Was he mad? Was he blind? If this was one of his 'strange mistakes', it was the strangest mistake I had ever come across.

I helped him on with his shoe (his foot), to avoid further complication. Dr P. himself seemed untroubled, indifferent, maybe amused. I resumed my examination. His visual acuity was good: he had no difficulty seeing a pin on the floor, though sometimes he missed it if it was placed to his left.

He saw all right, but what did he see? I opened out a copy of the *National Geographic Magazine*, and asked him to describe some pictures in it.

His responses here were very curious. His eyes would dart from one thing to another, picking up tiny features, individual features, as they had done with my face. A striking brightness, a colour, a shape would arrest his attention and elicit comment—but in no case did he get the scene-as-a-whole. He failed to see the whole, seeing only details, which he spotted like blips on a radar screen. He never entered into relation with the picture as a whole—never faced, so to speak, *its* physiognomy. He had no sense whatever of a landscape or scene.

Richard Wagner
1813–1883
What is Normality?
From *a Letter to August Roeckel*

26 January 1854

. . . In order to become a radically healthy human being, I went two years ago to a Hydropathic Establishment; I was prepared to give up Art and everything if I could once more become a child of Nature. But, my good friend, I was obliged to laugh at my own *naïveté* when I found myself almost going mad. None of us will reach the promised land—we shall all die in the wilderness. Intellect is, as someone has said, a sort of disease; it is incurable. In the present conditions of life, Nature only admits of abnormalities. At the best we can only hope to be martyrs; to refuse this vocation is to put oneself in opposition to the possibilities of life. For myself, I can no longer exist except as an artist; since I cannot compass love and life, all else repels me, or only interests me in so far as it has a bearing on Art. The result is a life of torment, but it is the only possible life. Moreover, some strange experiences have come to me through my works. When I think of the pain and discomfort which are now my chronic condition, I cannot but feel that my nerves are completely shattered: but marvellous to relate, on occasion, and under a happy stimulus, these nerves do wonders for me; a clearness of insight comes to me, and I experience a receptive and creative activity such as I have never known before. After this, can I say that my nerves are shattered? Certainly not. But I must admit that the normal condition of my temperament—as it has been developed through circumstances—is a state of exultation, whereas calm and repose is its abnormal condition. The fact is, it is only when I am 'beside myself' that I become my real self, and feel well and happy. . . .

(Translated from the German by Daphne Woodward)

Stendhal (Henri Beyle)
1783–1842

From *Life of Rossini*

In discussing the physical impact of music on the human system, Stendhal recounts the evidence of Dr Cotugno, the most distinguished physician in Naples, who testified that many young women died of excitement brought on while enjoying Rossini's *Mose in Egitto*:

'I could quote you more than forty cases of brain-fever or of violent nervous convulsions among young ladies with an over-ardent passion for music, brought on exclusively by the Jews' Prayer in the third act, with its extraordinary change of key!'

William Blake
1757–1827

The Sick Rose

O ROSE, thou art sick!
The invisible worm
That flies in the night,
In the howling storm,

Has found out thy bed
Of crimson joy,
And his dark secret love
Does thy life destroy.

Robert Schumann
1810–1856
Letters to Klara Wieck

29 November 1837

. . . BUT as regards the whole of this dark side of my life, I would like some day to reveal to you a deep secret about a *serious emotional disorder* I once went through: but it would take a long time, and covers the years from the summer of 1833 onwards. All the same, you shall hear about it one day, and then you will have the key to all my behaviour, my whole strange character. . . .

Leipzig, 11 February 1838

. . . MY life did not really begin until I became clear as to myself and my talent, decided to devote myself to art, and turned all my strength in a definite direction. That is to say, in 1830. In those days you were just a strange, headstrong little girl with a pair of beautiful eyes and a passion for cherries. . . . A few years went by. And already, in 1833, I began to be attacked by a melancholy that I avoided trying to account for; it came from the disappointment every artist feels when things do not go as quickly as he had hoped they would. I found little appreciation, and then came the loss of my right hand for playing. Then, amid all these gloomy thoughts and visions, only yours used to cheer me; indeed, without meaning or knowing it, you alone kept me all the long years from any association with women. As long ago as that I may have had an inkling that you might even become my wife; but it was all still too far away in the future; however that may be, I loved you from the very first as deeply as went with our age. . . . During the night of 17 to 18 October 1833, I was suddenly visited by the most terrible thought that can possibly come to a human creature—the most terrible thought that heaven can send as a punishment—that of 'losing my reason'—it overpowered me so violently that all comfort, all recourse to prayer, was silenced and turned to derision. But the anguish drove me from place to place—my breath failed me at the thought, 'suppose you lost the power to think'—Klara, anyone who was once reduced to that need fear no suffering, no sickness, no despair. . . .

(Translated from the German by Daphne Woodward)

Klara Schumann
1819–1896
From *Diary*

10 February 1854. THROUGHOUT the night Robert had such terrible sounds in his ears that he couldn't sleep for a single minute. First there was a continuous drone on one note, then an occasional second note as well. During the day it eased off. The next night was just as bad, and the following day as well—he had a mere two hours respite in the early morning, and at ten it all came back afresh. He is in terrible agony. Every sound he hears turns to music—music played on glorious-sounding instruments, he says, more beautiful than any music ever heard on earth. It utterly exhausts him. The doctor says there is nothing he can do.

17 February. In the night, not long after we had gone to bed, Robert got up and wrote down a melody which, he said, the angels had sung to him. Then he lay down again and talked deliriously the whole night, staring at the ceiling all the time. When morning came, the angels transformed themselves into devils and sang horrible music, telling him he was a sinner and that they were going to cast him into hell. He became hysterical, screaming in agony that they were pouncing on him like tigers and hyaenas, and seizing him in their claws. The two doctors who luckily came only just managed to control him.

(Translated from the German by Daphne Woodward)

Hector Berlioz
1803–1869
Letters on the 'Spleen'

Rome, 14 September 1831

. . . To tell you a word of myself by the way, I have nothing to talk about except the unspeakable boredom that is killing me, sapping my strength, eating me away, stifling me, choking me. . . . This town has no music, no theatre, no books, and when I am minded to escape from my habitual occupations, I do not know what to do with myself.

In fact the 'spleen' to which, as you know, I am so liable, has never before shown itself in such hideous guise; I can feel myself becoming as savage and violent as a madman. . . .

From *a Letter to Gasparo Spontini*

Rome, 29 March 1852

. . . You are too skilled at distinguishing between truth and falsehood to entertain a moment's doubt regarding my feelings towards the great man whose very name brings the flush of enthusiasm to my cheeks. The perpetual agitation in which I have been living, the heartbreak, the storms of every kind that have thundered over me for the past year, must serve as my excuse. I have hardly ever been in Rome for two months at a time, constantly hurrying off to Florence, Genoa, Nice, or Naples, on foot across the mountains, with no other aim than to tire myself, distract my mind and more easily resist the 'spleen' that was tormenting me. It would be tedious for you to learn the causes of the moral sickness from which I am by no means cured as yet. My existence up to now has been a strange, romantic tissue of adventures and distressing emotions, in which the latest episode is not the least. You may perhaps remember trying to dissuade me from a marriage I was about to contract while you were in Paris. Your advice, the soundness of which I now recognize, would have been useless and powerless against love; that was destroyed, a month after my departure, by the unfaithfulness of her who had inspired it. I now perceive the full extent of the danger I escaped, and congratulate myself upon my freedom with transports of delight. . . .

(Translated from the French by Daphne Woodward)

Alexander Borodin
1833–1887

Letter to His Wife on Mussorgsky's Alcoholism

25 October 1873

BY the way, here is some news for you: *Boris* [Mussorgsky's opera *Boris Godunov*] is to be given in its entirety. Gedeonov, when he returned from abroad to St Petersburg, as soon as he got out of the railway carriage, said in his first words to Lukashevich: 'Stage *Boris* without fail and as quickly as possible; send the score to Ferrero, I will order it passed.' Now they are already copying the parts. . . . And here is pitiful and sorrowful news: of the author of *Boris*. He has been drinking heavily. Nearly every day he sits in the Maldyaroslavetz restaurant on Morskaya, often drinking himself stiff. This summer the Sorokins saw him completely drunk in Pavlovsk; he caused a disturbance there; the affair reached the police. I have been told that he has already drunk himself to a state of seeing hallucinations and all sorts of trash. . . . This is horribly sad! Such a talented man and sinking so low morally. Now he periodically disappears, then reappears morose, untalkative, which is contrary to his usual habit. After a little while he again comes to himself—sweet, gay, amiable, and witty as ever. Devil, what a pity!

(Translated from the Russian by J. Leyda)

Anonymous
19th century

Sonnet Found in a Deserted Madhouse

OH that my soul a marrow-bone might seize!
For the old egg of my desire is broken,
Spilled is the pearly white and spilled the yolk, and
As the mild melancholy contents grease
My path the shorn lamb baas like bumblebees.
Time's trashy purse is as a taken token
Or like a thrilling recitation, spoken
By mournful mouths filled full of mirth and cheese.

And yet, why should I clasp the earthful urn?
Or find the frittered fig that felt the fast?
Or choose to chase the cheese around the churn?
Or swallow any pill from out the past?
Ah, no Love, not while your hot kisses burn
Like a potato riding on the blast.

John Clare
1793–1864

I Am

I AM: yet what I am none cares or knows,
    My friends forsake me like a memory lost;
I am the self-consumer of my woes,
    They rise and vanish in oblivious host,
Like shades in love and death's oblivion lost;
And yet I am, and live with shadows tost

Into the nothingness of scorn and noise,
    Into the living sea of waking dreams,
Where there is neither sense of life nor joys,
    But the vast shipwreck of my life's esteems;
And een the dearest—that I loved the best—
Are strange—nay, rather stranger than the rest.

I long for scenes where man has never trod;
    A place where woman never smiled or wept;
There to abide with my Creator, GOD,
    And sleep as I in childhood sweetly slept:
Untroubling and untroubled where I lie;
The grass below—above the vaulted sky.

Jon Silkin
1930–

Death of a Son

(who died in a mental hospital aged one)

SOMETHING has ceased to come along with me.
Something like a person: something very like one.
And there was no nobility in it
Or anything like that.

Something was there like a one year
Old house, dumb as stone. While the near buildings
Sang like birds and laughed
Understanding the pact

They were to have with silence. But he
Neither sang nor laughed. He did not bless silence
Like bread, with words.
He did not forsake silence.

But rather, like a house in mourning
Kept the eye turned in to watch the silence while
The other houses like birds
Sang around him.

And the breathing silence neither
Moved nor was still.

I have seen stones: I have seen brick
But this house was made up of neither bricks nor stone
But a house of flesh and blood
With flesh of stone

And bricks for blood. A house
Of stones and blood in breathing silence with the other
Birds singing crazy on its chimneys.
But this was silence,

This was something else, this was
Hearing and speaking though he was a house drawn
      Into silence, this was
          Something religious in his silence,

    Something shining in his quiet,
This was different this was altogether something else:
     Though he never spoke, this
        Was something to do with death.

    And then slowly the eye stopped looking
Inward. The silence rose and became still.
The look turned to the outer place and stopped,
      With the birds still shrilling around him.
        And as if he could speak

He turned over on his side with his one year
Red as a wound
He turned over as if he could be sorry for this
And out of his eyes two great tears rolled, like stones, and he died.

Wilfred Owen
1893–1918

Mental Cases

Who are these? Why sit they here in twilight?
Wherefore rock they, purgatorial shadows,
Drooping tongues from jaws that slob their relish,
Baring teeth that leer like skulls' teeth wicked?
Stroke on stroke of pain,—but what slow panic,
Gouged these chasms round their fretted sockets?
Ever from their hair and through their hands' palms
Misery swelters. Surely we have perished
Sleeping, and walk hell; but who these hellish?

—These are men whose minds the Dead have ravished.
Memory fingers in their hair of murders,
Multitudinous murders they once witnessed.
Wading sloughs of flesh these helpless wander,
Treading blood from lungs that had loved laughter.
Always they must see these things and hear them,
Batter of guns and shatter of flying muscles,
Carnage incomparable, and human squander,
Rucked too thick for these men's extrication.

Therefore still their eyeballs shrink tormented
Back into their brains, because on their sense
Sunlight seems a blood-smear; night comes blood-black;
Dawn breaks open like a wound that bleeds afresh.
—Thus their heads wear this hilarious, hideous,
Awful falseness of set-smiling corpses.
—Thus their hands are plucking at each other;
Picking at the rope-knouts of their scourging;
Snatching after us who smote them, brother,
Pawing us who dealt them war and madness.

F. W. Nietzsche
1844–1900

Collective Insanity

INSANITY in individuals is something rare—but in groups, parties, nations, and epochs it is the rule.

(From *Beyond Good and Evil*, (1886). *Translated from the German by
R. J. Hollingdale*)

⊰3⊱

Doctors and Psychiatrists

*D*ESCRIPTIONS *of doctors and their doings abound in all the arts. Some are highly flattering. For example, Robert Louis Stevenson (1850–94) in the Dedication which prefaces his poems expresses the view (and he had good reason to know) that the physician is the flower of our civilization.*

> Generosity he has, such as is possible to those who practise an art, never to those who drive a trade; discretion, tested by a hundred secrets; tact, tried in a thousand embarrassments; and what are more important, Heraclean cheerfulness and courage. So it is that he brings air and cheer into the sickroom, and often enough, though not so often as he wishes, brings healing.

Such sentiments are not universally shared. Some portraits are touched with irony—as the well-known description by Chaucer in the Preface to The Canterbury Tales—*and others are engraved with acid, as Shaw's account in his Preface to* The Doctor's Dilemma. *But, however they respond, thinkers and writers and artists have always been fascinated by doctors and the art of medicine. The same ambivalence is found in the treatment of the doctors of the soul (as Maimonides calls them), the psychiatrists.*

At the heart of medicine is the doctor–patient relationship with its peculiar mystique. The desirable side of this can be seen in T. S. Eliot's Cocktail Party, *but mystique easily turns into showmanship, quackery and (not necessarily undesirable) the 'alternative' forms of healing so common today. The words of 'The Doctor' are an example of the rumbustious side to medical life. The catchy tune makes the song easily adaptable for the ward party . . . The story of Dr James Barrie is extraordinary even in a male-dominated profession, and the case of Dr John Polidori illustrates that male doctors can also be extraordinary.*

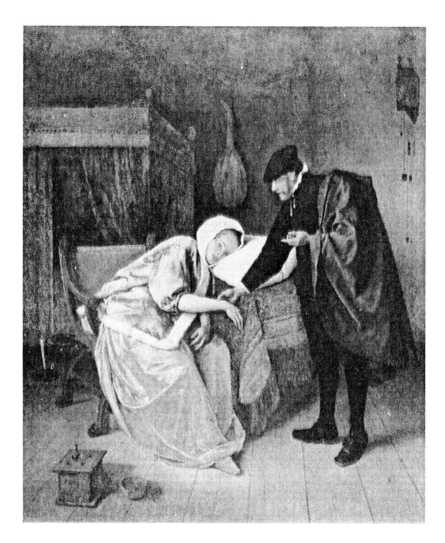

The Sick Woman (c. 1665). *Jan Steen.*
The taking of the pulse was emphasized in medical diagnosis from the time of Galen. But it was not until watches with minute hands became available, around 1700, that the pulse rate could be counted with any accuracy. Although the painter is clearly fascinated by the colours and textures of the clothes and tablecloth he also brings out the lethargy of the patient and the attentive concern of the doctor.

Some Ideals

Sir Thomas Browne
1605–1682

From *Religio Medici*

I FEEL not in me those sordid and unchristian desires of my profession; I do not secretly implore and wish for Plagues, rejoyce at Famines, revolve Ephemerides and Almanacks in expectation of malignant Aspects, fatal Conjunctions, and Eclipses. I rejoyce not at unwholesome Springs, nor unseasonable Winters: my Prayer goes with the Husbandman's; I desire every thing in its proper season, that neither men nor the times be put out of temper. Let me be sick myself, if sometimes the malady of my patient be not a disease unto me. I desire rather to cure his infirmities than my own necessities. Where I do him no good, methinks it is scarce honest gain; though I confess 'tis but the worthy salary of our well-intended endeavours. I am not only ashamed, but heartily sorry, that, besides death, there are diseases incurable: yet not for my own sake, or that they be beyond my Art, but for the general cause and sake of humanity, whose common cause I apprehend as mine own.

Terrence Hirst
1943–

The Widower

HE is younger than I realized,
I had always seen an old man
Creased and nicotine washed.

But still a star burst in the eyes
Which watched his trade die.
He stopped turning metal a decade ago,
Pressed his waistcoat, took a smaller pension.

How long since she died?, I'm thinking
As he cries without tears onto my desk.
Fifty bonded years and more,
Always speaking of her in the present tense.
Of course, she was his beautiful girl
In another generation's melody.
She waved him away to war,
Hugged him back, stroked away the melancholy.

So we sit out the allotted minutes,
Singing the old song of silence.
Faded silvering at the edge of an old mirror
Softening the mise-en-scene.
Two plotters deceiving even one another.
I cannot help him to bury her.
Perhaps next time we will come nearer.

George Eliot
1819–1880

From *Middlemarch*

AT present I have to make the new settler Lydgate better known to anyone interested in him than he could possibly be even to those who had seen the most of him since his arrival in Middlemarch. For surely all must admit that a man may be puffed and belauded, envied, ridiculed, counted upon as a tool and fallen in love with, or at least selected as a future husband, and yet remain virtually unknown—known merely as a cluster of signs for his neighbours' false suppositions. There was a general impression, however, that Lydgate was not altogether a common country doctor, and in Middlemarch at that time such an impression was significant of great things being expected from him. For everybody's family doctor was remarkably clever, and was understood to have immeasurable skill in the management and training of the most skittish or vicious diseases. The evidence of his cleverness was of the higher intuitive order, lying in his lady patients' immovable conviction, and was unassailable by any objection except that their intuitions were opposed by others equally strong; each lady who saw medical truth in Wrench and 'the strengthening treatment' regarding Toller and 'the lowering system' as medical perdition. For the heroic times of copious bleeding and blistering had not yet departed, still less the times of thorough-going theory, when disease in general was called by some bad name, and treated accordingly without shilly-shally—as if, for example, it were to be called insurrection, which must not be fired on with blank-cartridge, but have its blood drawn at once. The strengtheners and the lowerers were all 'clever' men in somebody's opinion, which is really as much as can be said for any living talents. Nobody's imagination had gone so far as to conjecture that Mr Lydgate could know as much as Dr Sprague and Dr Minchin, the two physicians, who alone could offer any hope when danger was extreme, and when the smallest hope was worth a guinea. Still I repeat, there was a general impression that Lydgate was something rather more uncommon than any general practitioner in Middlemarch. And this was true. He was but 27, an age at which many men are not quite common—at which they are hopeful of achievement, resolute in avoidance, thinking that Mammon shall never put a bit in their mouths and get astride their backs, but rather that Mammon, if they have anything to do with him, shall draw their chariot.

He had been left an orphan when he was fresh from a public school. His father, a military man, had made but little provision for three children, and when the boy Tertius asked to have a medical education, it seemed easier to his guardians to grant his request by apprenticing him to a country practitioner than to make any objections on the score of family dignity. He was one of the rarer lads who early get a decided bent and make up their minds that there is something particular in life which they would like to do for its own sake, and not because their fathers did it. Most of us who turn to any subject we love remember some morning or evening hour when we got on a high stool to reach down an untried volume, or sat with parted lips listening to a new talker, or for very lack of books began to listen to the voices within, as the first traceable beginning of our love. Something of that sort happened to Lydgate. He was a quick fellow, and when hot from play, would toss himself in a corner, and in five minutes be deep in any sort of book that he could lay his hands on: if it were Rasselas or Gulliver, so much the better, but Bailey's Dictionary would do, or the Bible with the Apocrypha in it. Something he must read, when he was not riding the pony, or running and hunting, or listening to the talk of men. All this was true of him at 10 years of age; he had then read through *Chrysal, or the Adventures of a Guinea,* which was neither milk for babes, nor any chalky mixture meant to pass for milk, and it had already occurred to him that books were stuff, and that life was stupid. His school studies had not much modified that opinion, for though he 'did' his classics and mathematics, he was not pre-eminent in them. It was said of him, that Lydgate could do anything he liked, but he had certainly not yet liked to do anything remarkable. He was a vigorous animal with a ready understanding, but no spark had yet kindled in him an intellectual passion; knowledge seemed to him a very superficial affair, easily mastered: judging from the conversation of his elders, he had apparently got already more than was necessary for mature life. Probably this was not an exceptional result of expensive teaching at that period of short-waisted coats, and other fashions which have not yet recurred. But, one vacation, a wet day sent him to the small home library to hunt once more for a book which might have some freshness for him: in vain! unless, indeed, he took down a dusty row of volumes with grey-paper backs and dingy labels—the volumes of an old Cyclopaedia which he had never disturbed. It would at least be a novelty to disturb them. They were on the highest shelf, and he stood on a chair to get them down. But he opened the volume which he first took from the shelf: somehow, one is apt to read in a makeshift attitude, just where it might seem inconvenient to do so. The page he opened on was under the heading of Anatomy, and the first passage that drew his eyes was on the valves of the heart. He was not much acquainted with valves of any sort, but he knew that *valvae* were folding doors, and through this crevice came a sudden light startling him with his first vivid notion of finely adjusted mechanism in the human frame. A liberal education had of course left him free to read the indecent passages in the school classics, but beyond a general sense of secrecy and obscenity in connection with his internal structure, had left his imagination quite unbiassed, so that for anything he knew his brains lay in small bags at his temples, and he had no more thought of representing to himself how his blood circulated than how paper served instead of gold. But the moment of vocation had come, and before he got down from his chair, the world was made new to him by a presentiment of endless processes filling the vast spaces planked out of his sight by that wordy ignorance which he had supposed to be knowledge. From that hour Lydgate felt the growth of an intellectual passion.

We are not afraid of telling over and over again how a man comes to fall in love with a woman and be wedded to her, or else be fatally parted from her. Is it due to excess of poetry or of stupidity that we are never weary of describing what King

James called a woman's 'makdom and her fairnesse', never weary of listening to the twanging of the old Troubadour strings, and are comparatively uninterested in that other kind of 'makdom and fairnesse' which must be wooed with industrious thought and patient renunciation of small desires? In the story of this passion, too, the development varies: sometimes it is the glorious marriage, sometimes frustration and final parting. And not seldom the catastrophe is bound up with the other passion, sung by the Troubadours. For in the multitude of middle-aged men who go about their vocations in a daily course determined for them much in the same way as the tie of their cravats, there is always a good number who once meant to shape their own deeds and alter the world a little. The story of their coming to be shapen after the average and fit to be packed by the gross, is hardly ever told even in their consciousness; for perhaps their ardour in generous unpaid toil cooled as imperceptibly as the ardour of other youthful loves, till one day their earlier self walked like a ghost in its old home and made the new furniture ghastly. Nothing in the world more subtle than the process of their gradual change! In the beginning they inhaled it unknowingly; you and I may have sent some of our breath towards infecting them, when we uttered our conforming falsities or drew our silly conclusions: or perhaps it came with the vibrations from a woman's glance.

Lydgate did not mean to be one of those failures, and there was the better hope of him because his scientific interest soon took the form of a professional enthusiasm: he had a youthful belief in his bread-winning work, not to be stifled by that initiation in makeshift called his 'prentice days; and he carried to his studies in London, Edinburgh, and Paris, the conviction that the medical profession as it might be was the finest in the world; presenting the most perfect interchange between science and art; offering the most direct alliance between intellectual conquest and the social good. Lydgate's nature demanded this combination: he was an emotional creature, with a flesh-and-blood sense of fellowship which withstood all the abstractions of special study. He cared not only for 'cases', but for John and Elizabeth, especially Elizabeth.

Walt Whitman
1819–1892

From *The Wound-Dresser*

Bearing the bandages, water and sponge,
Straight and swift to the wounded I go,
Where they lie on the ground after the battle brought in,
Where their priceless blood reddens the grass the ground,
Or to the rows of the hospital tent, or under the roof'd hospital,
To the long rows of cots up and down each side I return,
To each and all one after another I draw near, not one do I miss,
An attendant follows holding a tray, he carries a refuse pail,
Soon to be fill'd with clotted rags and blood, emptied, and fill'd again.

I onward go, I stop,
With hinged knees and steady hand to dress wounds,
I am firm with each, the pangs are sharp yet avoidable,
One turns to me his appealing eyes—poor boy! I never knew you,
Yet I think I could not refuse this moment to die for you, if that would save
    you.

On, I go, (open doors of time! open hospital doors!)
The crush'd head I dress (poor crazed hand tear not the bandage away,)
The neck of the cavalry-man with the bullet through and through I examine,
Hard the breathing rattles, quite glazed already the eye, yet life struggles hard,
(Come sweet death! be persuaded O beautiful death!
In mercy come quickly.)

From the stump of the arm, the amputated hand,
I undo the clotted lint, remove the slough, wash off the matter and blood,
Back on his pillow the soldier bends with curv'd neck and side-falling head,
His eyes are closed, his face is pale, he dares not look on the bloody stump,
And has not yet look'd on it.

I dress a wound in the side, deep, deep,
But a day or two more, for see the frame all wasted and sinking,
And the yellow-blue countenance see.

I dress a perforated shoulder, the foot with the bullet-wound
Cleanse the one with a gnawing and putrid gangrene, so sickening, so
  offensive,
While the attendant stands behind me aside me holding the tray and pail.

I am faithful, I do not give out,
The fractur'd thigh, the knee, the wound in the abdomen,
These and more I dress with impassive hand, (yet deep in my breast a fire, a
  burning flame.)

John Berger
1926–
Jean Mohr
1925–

From *A Fortunate Man: The Story of a Country Doctor*

HE is acknowledged as a good doctor. The organization of his practice, the facilities he offers, his diagnostic and clinical skill are probably somewhat underrated. His patients may not realize how lucky they are. But in a sense this is inevitable. Only the most self-conscious consider it lucky to have their elementary needs met. And it is on a very basic, elementary level that he is judged a good doctor.

They would say that he was straight, not afraid of work, easy to talk to, not stand-offish, kind, understanding, a good listener, always willing to come out when needed, very thorough. They would also say that he was moody, difficult to understand when on one of his theoretical subjects like sex, capable of doing things just to shock, unusual.

How he actually answers their needs as a doctor is far more complicated than any of these epithets imply. To understand this we must first consider the special character and depth of any doctor–patient relationship.

The primitive medicine-man, who was often also priest, sorcerer, and judge, was the first specialist to be released from the obligation of procuring food for the tribe. The magnitude of this privilege and of the power which it gave him is a direct reflection of the importance of the needs he served. An awareness of illness is part of the price that man first paid and still pays for his self-consciousness. This awareness increases the pain or disability. But the self-consciousness of which it is the result is a social phenomenon and so with this self-consciousness arises the possibility of treatment, of medicine.

We cannot imaginatively reconstruct the subjective attitude of a tribesman to his treatment. But within our culture today what is our own attitude? How do we acquire the necessary trust to submit ourselves to the doctor?

We give the doctor access to our bodies. Apart from the doctor, we only grant such access voluntarily to lovers—and many are frightened to do even this. Yet the doctor is a comparative stranger.

The degree of intimacy implied by the relationship is emphasized by the concern of all medical ethics (not only ours) to make an absolute distinction between the roles of doctor and lover. It is usually assumed that this is because the doctor can see women naked and can touch them where he likes and that this may sorely tempt him to make love to them. It is a crude assumption, lacking imagination. The conditions under which a doctor is likely to examine his patients are always sexually discouraging.

The emphasis in medical ethics on sexual correctness is not so much to restrict the doctor as to offer a promise to the patient: a promise which is far more than a reassurance that he or she will not be taken advantage of. It is a positive promise of physical intimacy without a sexual basis. Yet what can such intimacy mean? Surely it belongs to the experiences of childhood. We submit to the doctor by quoting to ourselves a state of childhood and simultaneously extending our sense of family to include him. We imagine him as an honorary member of the family.

In cases where the patient is fixated on a parent, the doctor may become a substitute for this parent. But in such a relationship the high degree of sexual content creates difficulties. In illness we ideally imagine the doctor as an elder brother or sister.

Something similar happens at death. The doctor is the familiar of death. When we call for a doctor, we are asking him to cure us and to relieve our suffering, but, if he cannot cure us, we are also asking him to witness our dying. The value of the witness is that he has seen so many others die. (This, rather than the prayers and last rites, was also the real value which the priest once had.) He is the living intermediary between us and the multitudinous dead. He belongs to us and he has belonged to them. And the hard but real comfort which they offer through him is still that of fraternity.

It would be a great mistake to 'normalize' what I have just said by concluding that quite naturally the patient wants a *friendly* doctor. His hopes and demands, however contradicted by previous experience, however protected they may be by scepticism, however undeclared even to himself, are much more profound and precise.

In illness many connections are severed. Illness separates and encourages a distorted, fragmented form of self-consciousness. The doctor, through his relationship with the invalid and by means of the special intimacy he is allowed, has to compensate for these broken connections and reaffirm the social content of the invalid's aggravated self-consciousness.

When I speak of a fraternal relationship—or rather of the patient's deep, unformulated expectation of fraternity—I do not of course mean that the doctor can or should behave like an actual brother. What is required of him is that he should recognize his patient with the certainty of an ideal brother. The function of fraternity is recognition. This individual and closely intimate recognition is required on both a physical and psychological level. On the former it constitutes the art of diagnosis. Good general diagnosticians are rare, not because most doctors lack medical knowledge, but because most are incapable of taking in all the possibly relevant facts—emotional, historical, environmental as well as physical. They are searching for specific conditions instead of the truth about a man which may then suggest various conditions. It may be that computers will soon diagnose better than doctors. But the facts fed to the computers will still have to be the result of intimate, individual recognition of the patient.

On the psychological level recognition means support. As soon as we are ill, we fear that our illness is unique. We argue with ourselves and rationalize, but a ghost of the fear remains. And it remains for a very good reason. The illness, as an undefined force, is a potential threat to our very being and we are bound to be highly conscious of the uniqueness of that being. The illness, in other words, shares in our own uniqueness. By fearing its threat, we embrace it and make it specially our own. That is why patients are inordinately relieved when doctors give their complaint a name. The name may mean very little to them; they may understand nothing of what it signifies; but because it has a name, it has an independent existence from them. They can now struggle or complain *against* it. To have a complaint recognized, that is to say defined, limited and depersonalized, is to be made stronger.

Maimonides
1135–1204
Physicians of the Soul

WHAT is the remedy for those whose souls are sick? Let them go to the wise men—who are physicians of the soul—and they will cure their disease by means of the character traits that they shall teach them, until they make them return to the middle way. Solomon said about those who recognize their bad character traits and do not go to the wise men to be cured: 'Fools despise admonition.'

(From *Laws Concerning Character Traits*, Chap. 2. *Translated from the Hebrew by Shlomo Pines*)

T. S. Eliot
1888–1965

From *The Cocktail Party*, II

[*A Consultation*]

[DR] REILLY. You have reason to believe that you are very ill?

EDWARD. I should have thought a doctor could see that for himself.
　　Or at least that he would enquire about the symptoms.
　　Two people advised me recently,
　　Almost in the same words, that I ought to see a doctor.
　　They said—again, in almost the same words—
　　That I was on the edge of a nervous breakdown.
　　I didn't know it then myself—but if they saw it
　　I should have thought that a doctor could see it.

REILLY. 'Nervous breakdown' is a term I never use.
　　It can mean almost anything.

EDWARD. And since then, I have realized
　　That mine is a very unusual case.

REILLY. All cases are unique, and very similar to others.

EDWARD. Is there a sanatorium to which you send such patients
    As myself, under your personal observation?

REILLY. You are very impetuous, Mr Chamberlayne.
    There are several kinds of sanatoria
    For several kinds of patient. And there are also patients
    For whom a sanatorium is the worst place possible.
    We must first find out what is wrong with you
    Before we decide what to do with you.

EDWARD. I doubt if you have ever had a case like mine.
    I have ceased to believe in my own personality.

REILLY. Oh, dear yes; this is serious. A very common malady.
    Very prevalent indeed.

EDWARD. I remember, in my childhood . . .

REILLY. I always begin from the immediate situation
    And then go back as far as I find necessary.
    You see, your memories of childhood—
    I mean, in your present state of mind—
    Would be largely fictitious; and as for your dreams,
    You would produce amazing dreams to oblige me.
    I could make you dream any kind of dream I suggested,
    And it would only go to flatter your vanity
    With the temporary stimulus of feeling interesting.

EDWARD. But I am obsessed by the thought of my own insignificance.

REILLY. Precisely. And I could make you feel important,
    And you would imagine it a marvellous cure;
    And you would go on, doing such amount of mischief
    As lay within your power—until you came to grief.
    Half of the harm that is done in this world
    Is due to people who want to feel important.

They don't mean to do harm—but the harm does not interest them.
Or they do not see it, or they justify it
Because they are absorbed in the endless struggle
To think well of themselves.

EDWARD. I must have done a great deal of harm.

REILLY. Oh, not so much as you would like to think:
Only, shall we say, within your modest capacity.

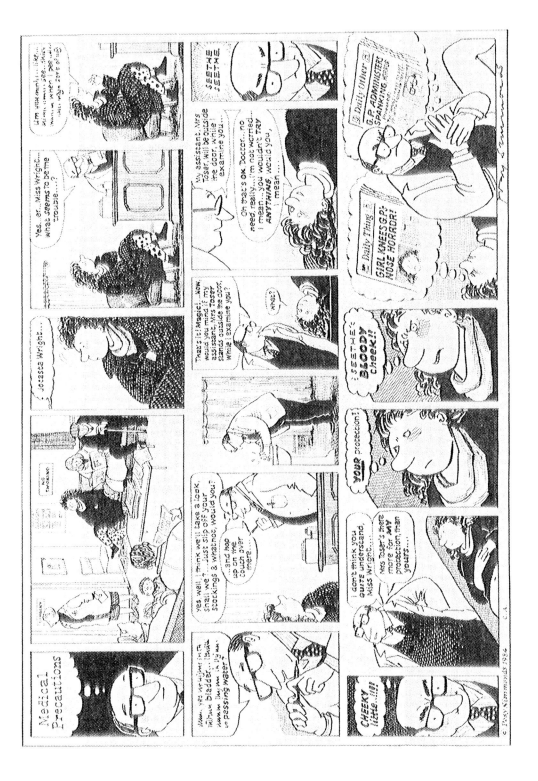

Less than Ideal

Geoffrey Chaucer
c.1340–1400

From *Prologue to The Canterbury Tales*

[*A Doctor of Medicine*]
WITH us ther was a Doctour of Physik:
In al this world ne was ther noon him lik
To speken of physik and of surgerye.
For he was grounded in astronomye.
He kepte his pacient a ful greet deel
In houres by his magik naturel.
Wel coude he fortunen the ascendent
Of his images for his pacient.
He knew the cause of every maladye,
Were it of hoot or cold or moiste or drye,
And where engendred and of what humour:
He was a verray parfit praktisour.
The cause yknowe, and of his harm the roote,
Anoon he yaf the sike man his boote.
Ful redy hadde he his apothecaries
To senden him drogges and his letuaries,
For eech of hem made other for to winne:
Hir frendshipe was nought newe to biginne.
Wel knew he the olde Esculapius,

And Deiscorides and eek Rufus,
Olde Ipocras, Hali, and Galien,
Serapion, Razis, and Avicen,
Averrois, Damascien, and Constantin,
Bernard, and Gatesden, and Gilbertin.
Of his diete mesurable was he,
For it was of no superfluitee,
But of greet norissing and digestible.
His studye was but litel on the Bible.
In sanguin and in pers he clad was al,
Lined with taffata and with sendal;
And yit he was but esy of dispence;
He kepte that he wan in pestilence.
For gold in physik is a cordial,
Therfore he loved gold in special.

Physik] medicine	boote] remedy	pers] blue
For] because	drogges] drugs	sendal] silk
astronomye] astrology	letuaries] medicines	dispence] expenditure
kepte] tended to	mesurable] moderate	pestilence] plague
deel] closely	norissing] nourishment	For] because
praktisour] practitioner	sanguin] blood-red	cordial] stimulant
yknowe] known		

Franz Schubert
1797–1828

To His Friends in Vienna

Zseliz, 8 September 1818

Dear Schober,   Dear Senn,
Dear Spaun   Dear Streinsberg,
Dear Mayrhofer,   Dear Wayss,
                Dear Weidlich,

. . . I WAS attending an auction of cows and oxen when your fat letter was handed to
me. I broke the seal, and gave a loud cry of joy when I saw the name of Schober. . . .
No one here has any feeling for true art, except (if I am not mistaken) the Countess
now and then. So I am alone with my beloved, and must conceal her in my room, in

my piano, in my bosom. Though this often grieves me, on the other hand it elevates me in proportion. So do not be afraid that I shall stay away any longer than is strictly necessary. Meanwhile, I have produced several songs, which I hope have turned out very well. . . .

Our castle is not particularly large, but built in a very elegant style. It stands in a beautiful garden. I am lodged in the estate manager's house. It is fairly quiet, except for about 40 geese, which sometimes strike up such a chorus of cackling that one cannot hear oneself speak. The people here are all most kindly. It is rare to find an aristocrat's household living in such harmony as this one. The estate manager, a Slavonian, is a worthy man with a high opinion of his erstwhile talent for music. Even now he can play two German dances in 3/4 time on the lute like a virtuoso. His son, who is a philosophy student, has just arrived for the holidays, I should like to make friends with him. His wife is like all women who wish to be thought genteel. The comptroller is the right man in the right place, with a shrewd eye for his pockets and money-bags. The doctor is really clever, but though only 24 he is as fussy about his health as an old lady. Something most unnatural there. The surgeon is my favourite, a respectable old man of 75, always serene and cheerful. May God grant us all such a happy old age. The Justice is a very natural, worthy man. One of the Count's companions, a merry old fellow and a good musician, often comes to keep me company. The cook, the lady's maid, the housemaid, the children's nurse, the steward, etc., and the 2 equerries, are all pleasant people. The cook is somewhat dissolute, the lady's maid 30 years old, the housemaid very pretty, often keeps me company.

(Translated from the German by Daphne Woodward)

Frédéric Chopin
1810–1849

From *a Letter to Julien Fontana in Paris*

Palma, 3 December 1838

My Julien,

I HAVE been as sick as a dog for the last fortnight. I had caught cold in spite of the eighteen degrees centigrade, the roses, the orange-trees, the palms, and the fig-trees. Three doctors—the most celebrated on this island—examined me. One of them sniffed at my spittle, another tapped to find out where I spat it from, the third felt me, listening how I spat. The first said I was going to die, the second that I was actually dying, the third that I was dead already. . . . I had great difficulty in escaping from their bleedings, vesicatories, and pack-sheets, but thanks be to providence, I am myself again. But my illness was unfavourable to the *Preludes*, which will reach you God knows when. In a few days' time I am moving to the most beautiful place in the world; I shall have the sea, the mountains, everything you can imagine. I am to live in an old monastery, huge and deserted, from which Mend[izabal] seems to have expelled the Carthusians for my benefit. It is near Palma and nothing could be more beautiful. There are arcades, the most poetic cemetery, in short I shall be comfortable there. . . .

(Translated from the French by Daphne Woodward)

Anton Chekhov
1860–1904
From *Ward 6*

DR RAGIN was a remarkable man in his way. He was said to have been very religious as a young man and to have thought of taking holy orders. On finishing his studies at the secondary school in 1863 he had intended to enter a theological college, but his father, a doctor of medicine and a surgeon, had poured scorn on his plans and had declared that he would disown him if he became a priest. How much of this was true I don't know, but I have often heard it said that he never felt any vocation for medicine or for any specialized branch of science.

Be that as it may, he did not take holy orders after graduating from the medical faculty. He showed no sign of religiosity, and was as little like a priest at the beginning of his medical career as he is now.

He looked like a heavily built, coarse-featured peasant; his face, beard, straight hair, and strong, ungainly build reminded one of an innkeeper on the highway— well fed, intemperate, and harsh. His stern face was covered with blue veins, his eyes were small, his nose red. Being very tall and broad-shouldered, he had enormous hands and feet; one blow with his fist and you would be as good as dead. Yet he walked softly, cautiously, insinuatingly; meeting someone in a narrow passage, he was the first to stop and give way, saying 'Sorry' not in a deep bass voice, as you might expect, but in a soft, thin treble. He had a small tumour on his neck which prevented him from wearing stiff starched collars, and that was why he always went about in soft linen or cotton shirts. He did not dress like a doctor at all. He wore the same suit for ten years, and when he did buy new clothes, which he usually bought at a Jewish shop, they looked just as worn and crumpled on him as the old suit; he received patients, dined, and paid visits in one and the same coat; he did it not because he was a miser but because he was completely indifferent to his personal appearance.

When Dr Ragin arrived in our town to take up his post, the 'charitable institution' was in an appalling state. It was quite impossible to breathe in the wards, the corridors, and the hospital yard for the stench. The male hospital attendants, the nurses, and their families slept in the wards together with the patients. Everybody complained that cockroaches, bedbugs, and lice made life in the hospital unbearable. The surgical ward was never free from erysipelas. In the whole hospital there were only two scalpels and not a single thermometer; the baths were used for storing potatoes. The superintendent, the matron, and the doctor's assistant robbed the patients, and of the old doctor, Ragin's predecessor, it was said that he had engaged in illegal sales of the hospital spirits and had kept a veritable harem recruited from the nurses and the female patients. In the town they knew perfectly well of the disgraceful goings-on in the hospital and exaggerated them, but it did not seem to worry anyone; some justified it by saying that it was after all only peasants and tradesmen who went to hospital and that they could not possibly be dissatisfied since they were much worse off at home. They did not expect to be fed on grouse, did they? Others argued that the town could not be expected to run a good hospital without assistance from the rural council; they ought to be grateful for any hospital, even a bad one. As for the rural council, which had only recently come into being, it did not open a hospital in the town or its vicinity on the ground that the town had one already.

After inspecting the hospital, Dr Ragin came to the conclusion that it was an immoral institution, highly detrimental to the health of those who lived in it. In his opinion the best thing to do was to discharge the patients and close down the hospital. But he realized that he had not the authority to do so, and that it would be no good, anyhow; for clearing away all the physical and moral uncleanliness from one place would merely transfer it to another; it was necessary to wait till it disappeared of itself. Besides, if people opened a hospital and kept it going, it meant that there was a need for it; prejudices and all sorts of foul and abominable things which one came across in life were necessary, for in the course of time they were converted into something useful, just as manure was converted into fertile black earth. There was nothing good on earth that had not originally had something vile in it.

Having taken up his duties, Dr Ragin seems to have regarded these abuses with apparent indifference. He merely asked the male hospital attendants and nurses not to spend the night in the wards and installed two cupboards of surgical instruments; the superintendent, the matron, the medical assistant, and the erysipelas stayed where they were.

Dr Ragin was a great believer in intelligence and honesty, but he lacked the strength of character and the confidence in his own right to assert himself in order to see to it that the life around him should be honest and intelligent. He simply did not know how to give orders, to prohibit, or to insist. It was almost as though he had taken a vow never to raise his voice or to use the imperative mood. He found it difficult to say 'Give me—' or 'Bring me—'. When he felt hungry, he cleared his throat irresolutely and said to his cook: 'I wonder if I could have a cup of tea. . . .' Or: 'I wonder if I could have my dinner now. . . .' But to tell the superintendent to stop stealing and give him the sack, or to abolish the unnecessary, parasitical office altogether, was quite beyond his strength. When deceived or flattered or handed a quite obviously fraudulent account for signature, he turned as red as a lobster and felt guilty, but he signed the account all the same; when the patients complained that they were not given enough to eat or that the nurses ill-treated them, he looked embarrassed and muttered guiltily: 'All right, all right, I'll look into it later. . . . I expect there must be some misunderstanding. . . .'

At first Dr Ragin worked very hard. He received patients everyday from morning till dinner-time, performed operations, and even did a certain amount of midwifery. Among the women he gained a reputation for being very conscientious and very good at diagnosing illnesses, especially those of women and children. But as time passed he got tired of the monotony and the quite obvious uselessness of his work. One day he would receive thirty patients, the next day thirty-five, the next day after that forty, and so on from day to day, from one year to another, though the death-rate in the town did not decrease and the patients continued to come. To give any real assistance to forty patients between morning and dinner-time was a physical impossibility, which meant that his work was a fraud, necessarily a fraud. He received twelve thousand out-patients in a given-year, which bluntly speaking meant that he had deceived twelve thousand people. To place the serious cases in the wards and treat them in accordance with the rules of science was also impossible, for although there were rules, there was no science; on the other hand, if he were to leave philosophy alone and follow the rules pedantically, like the other doctors, he would above all require cleanliness and fresh air and not filth, wholesome food and not stinking sour cabbage soup, good assistants and not thieves.

Besides, why prevent people dying if death was the normal and legitimate end of us all? Did it really matter if some huckster or government clerk lived an extra five or six years? And if the aim of the medical profession was to alleviate suffering by the administration of medicine, the question inevitably arose: why alleviate suffering? For in the first place it was argued that man could only achieve perfection through suffering, and, secondly, if mankind really learnt to alleviate suffering by pills and drops it would give up religion and philosophy, in which it had hitherto found not only protection from all misfortunes but even happiness. Pushkin suffered terribly before he died, and poor Heine lay paralysed for several years; why then should some Andrey Yefimych or a Matryona Savishna not be ill, particularly if but for suffering their lives would be as meaningless and insipid as the life of an amoeba?

Crushed by such arguments, Dr Ragin lost heart and stopped going to the hospital every day.

(Translated from the Russian by David Magarshak)

Showmen and Quacks

Galen
c. AD 129–c.200

A Case History

UPON the occasion of my first visit to Rome I completely won the admiration of the philosopher Glaucon by the diagnosis which I made in the case of one of his friends. Meeting me one day in the street he shook hands with me and said: 'I have just come from the house of a sick man, and I wish that you would visit him with me. He is a Sicilian physician, the same person with whom I was walking when you met me the other day.'

'What is the matter with him?' I asked.

Then coming nearer to me he said, in the frankest manner possible: 'Gorgias and Apelas told me yesterday that you had made some diagnoses and prognoses which looked to them more like acts of divination than products of the medical art pure and simple. I would therefore like very much to see some proof, not of your knowledge but of this extraordinary art which you are said to possess.'

At this very moment we reached the entrance of the patient's house, and so, to my regret, I was prevented from having any further conversation with him on the subject and from explaining to him how the element of good luck often renders it possible for a physician to give, as it were offhand, diagnoses and prognoses of this exceptional character. Just as we were approaching the first door, after entering the house, we met a servant who had in his hand a basin which he had brought from the sick room and which he was on his way to empty upon the dung heap. As we passed him I appeared not to pay any attention to the contents of the basin, but at a mere glance I perceived that they consisted of a thin sanio-sanguinolent fluid, in which floated excrementitious masses that resembled shreds of flesh—an unmistakable evidence of disease of the liver. Glaucon and I, not a word having been spoken by either of us, passed on into the patient's room. When I put out my hand to feel of the latter's pulse, he called my attention to the fact that he had just had a stool, and that, owing to the circumstance of his having gotten out of bed, his pulse might be accelerated. It was in fact somewhat more rapid than it should be, but I attributed this to the existence of an inflammation. Then, observing upon the window-sill a vessel containing a mixture of hyssop and honey and water, I made up my mind that the patient, who was himself a physician, believed that the malady from which he was suffering was a pleurisy; the pain which he experienced on the right side in the region of the false ribs (and which is also associated with inflammation of the liver) confirming him in this belief, and thus inducing him to order for the relief of the slight accompanying cough the mixture to which I have called attention. It was then that the idea came into my mind that, as fortune had thrown the opportunity in my way, I would avail myself of it to enhance my reputation in Glaucon's estimation.

Accordingly, placing my hand on the patient's right side over the false rib, I remarked: 'This is the spot where the disease is located.'

He, supposing that I must have gained this knowledge by simply feeling his pulse, replied with a look which plainly expressed admiration mingled with astonishment, that I was entirely right.

'And', I added simply to increase his astonishment, 'you will doubtless admit that at long intervals you feel impelled to indulge in a shallow, dry cough, unaccompanied by any expectoration.'

As luck would have it, he coughed in just this manner almost before I had got the words out of my mouth. At this Glaucon, who had hitherto not spoken a word, broke out into a volley of praises.

'Do not imagine,' I replied, 'that what you have observed represents the utmost of which the medical art is capable in the matter of fathoming the mysteries of disease in a living person. There still remain one or two other symptoms to which I will direct your attention.'

Turning then to the patient I remarked: 'When you draw a longer breath you feel a more marked pain, do you not, in the region which I indicated; and with this pain there is associated a sense of weight in the hypochondrium?'

At these words the patient expressed his astonishment and admiration in the strongest possible terms. I wanted to go a step farther and announce to my audience still another symptom which is sometimes observed in the more serious maladies of the liver (scirrhus, for example), but I was afraid that I might compromise the laudation which had been bestowed upon me. It then occurred to me that I might safely make this announcement if I put it somewhat in the form of a prognosis.

So I remarked to the patient: 'You will probably soon experience, if you have not already done so, a sensation of something pulling upon the right clavicle.'

He admitted that he had already noticed this symptom.

'Then I will give just one more evidence of this power of divination which you believe that I possess. You, yourself, before I arrived on the scene, had made up your mind that your ailment was an attack of pleurisy, etc.'

Glaucon's confidence in me and in the medical art, after this episode, was unbounded.

(From *De Locis Affectis*, Bk II. *Translated from the Latin by Logan Clendening*)

George Crabbe
1754–1832

From *The Borough*

BUT now our quacks are gamesters, and they play
With craft and skill to ruin and betray;
With monstrous promise they delude the mind,
And thrive on all that tortures human-kind.
　　Void of all honour, avaricious, rash,
The daring tribe compound their boasted trash—
Tincture or syrup, lotion, drop or pill;
All tempt the sick to trust the lying bill;
And twenty names of cobblers turn'd to squires,
Aid the bold language of these blushless liars.
There are among them those who cannot read,
And yet they'll buy a patent, and succeed;
Will dare to promise dying sufferers aid,—
For who, when dead, can threaten or upbraid?
With cruel avarice still they recommend
More draughts, more syrup, to the journey's end:

'I feel it not';—'Then take it every hour.'—
'It makes me worse';—'Why, then it shows its
    power.'—
'I fear to die';—'Let not your spirits sink,
'You're always safe, while you believe and drink.'
    How strange to add, in this nefarious trade,
That men of parts are dupes by dunces made:
That creatures nature meant should clean our streets
Have purchased lands and mansions, parks and seats;
Wretches with conscience so obtuse, they leave
Their untaught sons their parents to deceive;
And, when they're laid upon their dying-bed,
No thought of murder comes into their head;
Nor one revengeful ghost to them appears,
To fill the soul with penitential fears.

Thomas Hood
1798–1845

The Doctor

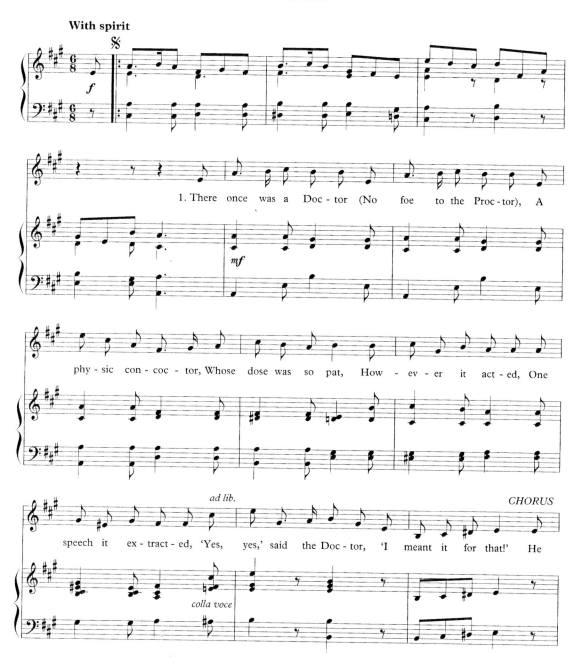

1. There once was a Doc - tor (No foe to the Proc - tor), A
phy - sic con - coc - tor, Whose dose was so pat, How - ev - er it act - ed, One
speech it ex - tract - ed, 'Yes, yes,' said the Doc - tor, 'I meant it for that!' He

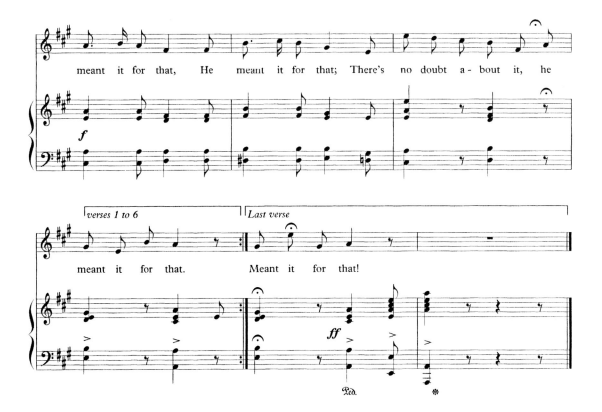

And first, all 'unaisy,'
Like woman that's crazy,
In flies Mrs Casey—
'Do come to poor Pat!
The blood's running faster!
He's torn off the plaster'—
'Yes, yes,' said the doctor,
'I meant it for that!'

Anon, with an antic
Quite strange and romantic,
A woman comes frantic—
'What could you be at?
My darling dear Alick
You've sent him oxalic!'
'Yes, yes,' said the doctor,
'I meant it for that!'

Then in comes another,
Despatched by his mother,
A blubbering brother
Who gives a rat-tat—
'Oh, poor little sister
Has licked off a blister!'
'Yes, yes,' said the doctor,
'I meant it for that!'

Now home comes the flunkey,
His own powder monkey,
But dull as a donkey—
With basket and that—
'The draught for the squire, sir,
He chucked in the fire, sir.'
'Yes, yes,' said the doctor,
'I meant it for that!'

The next is the pompous
Head-beadle, old Bumpus,
'Lord! here is a rumpus;
That pauper, old Nat,
In some drunken notion
Has drunk up his lotion.'
'Yes, yes,' said the doctor,
'I meant it for that!'

At last comes a servant,
In grief very fervent,
'Alas! Doctor Derwent,
Poor master is flat!
He's drawn his last breath, sir,
That dose was his death, sir.'
'Yes, yes,' said the doctor,
'I meant it for that!'

[Words by Thomas Hood, music by Ernest Newton]

A Woman in Medicine

Brian Hurwitz, General Practitioner
1951–
Ruth Richardson, Historian
1951–

Inspector-General James Barry MD: Putting the Woman in Her Place

JAMES BARRY qualified in medicine at the University of Edinburgh in 1812, at the age of only 17. Barry's MD thesis, in Latin, was on hernia of the groin. As its epigraph it had a quotation from the classical dramatist Menander, which urged the examiners: 'Do not consider my youth, but whether I show a man's wisdom.'

No one spotted the real meaning of these words, and Barry proceeded to walk the wards as a pupil dresser at the United Hospitals of Guy's and St Thomas's under the tutelage of Astley Cooper. In January 1813 Dr Barry was 'examined and passed as a Regimental Surgeon' by the Royal College of Surgeons of London. Thus began a career that was to span almost half a century and take in half the globe and was to culminate in the rank of inspector-general of hospitals in the British army.

A REVELATION

James Barry's life and career have since provided inspiration for several literary works, including biographies, at least four novels, and two plays. The cause of this interest is not difficult to find. This 'most skilful of physicians, and . . . most wayward of men' died at 14 Margaret Street, Marylebone, during the summer of 1865. Shortly afterwards the following report appeared in the *Manchester Guardian*:

An incident is just now being discussed in military circles so extraordinary that, were not the truth capable of being vouched for by official authority, the narration would certainly be deemed absolutely incredible. Our officers quartered at the Cape between fifteen and twenty years ago may remember a certain Dr Barry attached to the medical staff there, and enjoying a reputation for considerable skill in his profession, especially for firmness, decision and rapidity in difficult operations. This gentleman had entered the army in 1813, had passed, of course, through the grades of assistant surgeon and surgeon in various regiments, and had served as such in various quarters of the globe. His professional acquirements had procured for him promotion to the staff at the Cape. About 1840 he became promoted to be medical inspector, and was transferred to Malta. He proceeded from Malta to Corfu where he was quartered for many years . . . and upon his death was discovered to be a woman. The motives that occasioned, and the time when commenced this singular deception are both shrouded in mystery. But thus it stands as an indubitable fact, that a woman was for forty years an officer in the British service, and fought one duel and had sought many more, had pursued a legitimate medical education, and received a regular diploma, and had acquired almost a celebrity for skill as a surgical operator.

As a result of the article, the then Registrar General requested further information from the certifying doctor, David McKinnon, as to the truth of rumours concerning Barry's sex. McKinnon replied that he had not examined the body and had no 'purpose in making the discovery as I could positively swear to the identity of the body as being that of a person whom I had been acquainted with as Inspector General of Hospitals for a period of eight or nine years'. McKinnon had merely certified the cause of death as 'diarrhoea.' His reluctance to examine the corpse may be explained by the fact that Barry died during an epidemic. The local nurse who laid the body out had no such qualms and, as a result of a dispute concerning payment for her work, revealed the startling facts to Barry's army agents. There followed a confrontation at their office in St James's, which McKinnon described thus:

> The woman who performed the last offices for Dr Barry was waiting to speak to me. . . . Amongst other things she said that Dr Barry was a female and that I was a pretty Doctor not to know this, and that she would not like to be attended by me . . . she had examined the body and . . . it was a perfect female.

By this time the story had gained its own momentum, and the *Guardian*'s copy, which had itself originated in a Dublin newspaper, reappeared with additions in the *Medical Times and Gazette* under the title 'A female medical combatant'. The editor of the *British Medical Journal* also reprinted the story and commented, 'The gentleman alluded to was well known to many members of the profession. It was always suspected by those who knew him well in the army that he was a she.'

Within a week a denial appeared in the *Medical Times and Gazette*, which asserted, 'The stories which have been circulated . . . are too absurd to be gravely refuted.' The writer was a colleague who, like McKinnon, put forward what was to become an accepted apologia—that Barry *was* male or, if not, perhaps a hermaphrodite.

THE SECRET IS KEPT

The evidence, however, points in another direction. As a French medical journal commented at the time, 'the enshrouders themselves were mothers of families . . . who had seen, examined, and touched. Colleagues and patients throughout Barry's military career had noticed her feminine appearance and manner, and on at least one occasion Barry's sex was literally revealed. While she was seriously ill with yellow fever in Trinidad in 1841 two of her medical subordinates entered her sickroom to pry and, finding Barry asleep, turned back the bedclothes:

> At that moment the P.M.O. awoke to consciousness and gazed at us bewilderingly. But she quickly recovered presence of mind, and asked us in low tones to swear solemnly not to disclose her secret as long as she lived.

How Barry persuaded these men to respect her secret is not known, but this witness kept his silence for 15 years after Barry's death and revealed the discovery only after the publication of a novel about her life. *A Modern Sphinx* appeared in 1881 as a triple-decker novel. As a young man, its author, Ebenezer Rogers, had shared a cabin with Barry on board a Caribbean steamer: 'A goat was on board to provide her with milk; she was a strict vegetarian, and she was accompanied by a negro servant and a little dog.'

Throughout her career Barry used, with varying success, techniques to disguise her real sex, and Rogers came to appreciate only retrospectively that her behaviour had involved rituals of concealment as well as eccentricity. He recalled later in a letter to the *Lancet*: 'I well remember how in harsh and peevish voice, she ordered me out of the cabin—blow high, blow low—while she dressed in the morning. "Now then, youngster, clear out of my cabin while I dress," she would say.' Another colleague observed that Barry 'always took care never to be seen . . . like any ordinary man,' a reference to her need for privacy to conceal bodily functions.

At the same time, again with varying success, Barry asserted an apparent masculinity. In the Cape her shoulder pads gave rise to the sobriquet 'Kapok Doctor', and her oversized sword and spurs were the subject of comment. She adopted a seriousness of manner that many found off putting and was quick to take offence: 'He was always suspected of being a female from his effeminate features and voice, and having neither beard nor whiskers. He was a very bold person, and challenged one or two of our officials for naming him a diminutive creature.'

Barry's parentage remains a mystery. What is known suggests that she was probably the niece of the artist James Barry RA, whose name she adopted. Her two middle names, Miranda and Steuart, were taken from her influential sponsors, General Francisco de Miranda, a Venezuelan revolutionary patriot and scholar, and David Steuart Erskine, Lord Buchan, art collector and savant. Both men were close friends of the artist and enlightened supporters of female education. Barry acknowledged her debt to both men in the dedication to her MD thesis.

Just before Barry's birth Lord Buchan had written a series of essays in *The Bee*, a periodical designed for the edification and entertainment of young ladies. These essays were republished in book form in Edinburgh in 1812 while Barry was studying medicine there. Buchan's essay *On Female Education* argued that in denying women education, his countrymen were guilty of the cerebral equivalent of Chinese foot binding. Significantly, Buchan wrote several of these essays in the guise of a woman, signing them 'Sophia'.

Lord Buchan certainly gave his patronage to James Barry during her medical education and may have introduced her to influential friends in the army medical service. Ebenezer Rogers believed that she probably 'possessed . . . backdoor influence' as her promotion was rapid, and 'she even managed to jump up, two steps at a time, in her ambitious climb to the top of the tree.'

A REFORMING DOCTOR

But Barry's army service records a string of impressive achievements, which in themselves account for her advancement. Her army duties often extended beyond the confines of military medicine into the communities in which she served. As a surgeon she is credited with the first successful Caesarean section in South Africa in 1826—one of the earliest recorded cases in the world in which both mother and child survived. Barry conducted experiments into the medicinal value of local plants in treating syphilis and on preventing corrosion in pipes carrying fresh water. She received the personal thanks of the Duke of Wellington for her work in Malta during an outbreak of cholera in 1846 and was promoted shortly afterwards to deputy inspector-general.

In her colonial postings James Barry gained a formidable reputation as a doctor and administrator who challenged the power of local oligarchies and would not brook corrupt or negligent practices. She drew up clear and humane rules for treating inmates in the Cape leper colony, protested about brutality towards prisoners, and attempted to control the sale to the general public of spurious and dangerous medicines. On one occasion, to prevent an epidemic of sunstroke among men of the 71st Highland Light Infantry, she convened a medical board to declare its colonel *non compos mentis* for drilling the men in the midday sun. A soldier later recalled that the regiment subsequently embarked for the Crimea, followed by its colonel, 'who persistently applied to Lord Raglan to be restored to command. His services, however, were declined, much to the satisfaction of the men.' An officer later remarked: 'Although it is quite certain that for these ''interfering ways'' many of the senior officers disliked Barry, there must be still many officers and a great many of the ex-rank and file who remember her with gratitude.'

CONFLICT IN THE CRIMEA

At the outset of her army medical career Barry had been appointed physician to Raglan's brother Lord Charles Somerset, then governor of the Cape. She had saved the life of one of his daughters and had become a favourite with the family. Lord Raglan, then commander in chief of the British forces in the Crimea, thus had reason to respect her medical skill. Had Barry been appointed inspector-general of hospitals in the Crimea the medical history of the war might have been altogether different. Such a notion is not merely fanciful: the beleaguered incumbent of that office, Sir John Hall, confided to his diary late in 1854 his fears that Raglan wanted to 'get rid' of him to 'make room for his protégé Barry'. In fact Barry was fully occupied until the following autumn in Corfu supervising the treatment of 500 casualties from the Crimea. She had volunteered for the task and achieved a much lower mortality than was ever recorded in Scutari. In the mean time Raglan had died.

Barry took her annual leave in the Crimea in 1855. The senior medical officer at the Barrack Hospital in Scutari wrote to Hall to warn him of her imminent arrival:

> I may as well warn you that you are to have a visit from the renowned Dr Barry. He called upon me yesterday and as I never met him before his appearance and conversation rather surprised me. He appears to be in his dotage and is an intolerable bore. . . . He will expect you to listen to every quarrel he has had since coming into the Service. You probably know that they are not a few.

Perhaps unexpectedly Hall and Barry became friends. Later Hall sent Barry a copy of his *Observations* on the report of the Crimea Sanitary Commission, which had been orchestrated by Florence Nightingale and was highly critical of the army medical department. Barry's fierce loyalty to the service is evident in her supportive response to Hall's manuscript, as it was in her only known encounter with Florence Nightingale, which occurred in the Crimea. Nightingale was later to recall it with some bitterness:

> I never had such a blackguard rating in all my life—I who have had more than any woman—than from this Barry sitting on his horse, while I was crossing the Hospital Square with only my cap on in the sun. He kept me standing in the midst of quite a crowd of soldiers, Commissariat, servants, camp followers, etc., etc., every one of whom behaved like a gentleman during the scolding I received while (she) behaved like a brute. . . . After she was dead, I was told that (he) was a woman. . . . I should say that (she) was the most hardened creature I ever met.

A VALE OF TEARS

The careers of two extraordinary nineteenth-century women intersect at this point. Each had chosen a different path by which to transcend the limitations imposed upon her sex. Both had rejected traditional female social and familial roles. In 1855 both were women in a man's world whose chosen strategies reflected different ambitions: James Barry had joined an existing professional structure and achieved piecemeal reforms from within, Florence Nightingale had determined to create an entirely new structure. In the Crimea Barry could exercise rank and power over Nightingale, but she probably had little notion how profoundly her own future career would be affected by the younger 'lady with the lamp'. Florence Nightingale's determination to reform the army medical department, and her contempt for Sir John Hall, the next in line for promotion to director-general, resulted after much political chicanery in the appointment of Sir Thomas Alexander, then serving in Canada. Barry was sent out as his replacement, promoted to inspector-general of hospitals. She wrote to a colleague:

> So I am to go to Canada, to cool myself after such a long residence in the Tropics and Hot Countries. . . . This much for changes and chances in this 'World of woe, this Vale of Tears' as schollars say.

Nevertheless, Barry arrived in Canada with her old reforming zeal intact and, despite the freezing weather, set about improving soldiers' diet, accommodation, and water supplies. She recommended the establishment of separate quarters for married servicemen and recreational facilities such as libraries and athletics for all ranks. Barry was by now 64 years old and had worked for 40 years in the tropics. The Canadian winters affected her health, and in 1859 she caught influenza, developed bronchitis, and returned sick to London in a weak state.

Barry's Canadian physician, Dr G. W. Campbell, later became dean of McGill Medical School. His embarrassment at having failed to detect her sex, despite treating her for a chest complaint, was relished by his students, among them the young Osler, who later recalled that Campbell had told his class in mitigation:

> Gentlemen, if I had not stood in some awe of Inspector General Barry's rank and medical attainments, I would have examined him—that is, her—far more thoroughly. Because I did not and because his—confound it, her—bed-room was always in almost total darkness when I paid my calls, this, ah, crucial point escaped me.

On her return to London, Barry appeared before a medical board and was pronounced unfit for further service. Although she petitioned the Secretary of State for War, she was retired from the army medical service on half pay in July 1859, her sex still undiscovered.

(The fully referenced version of this article can be found in the *British Medical Journal*, **298** (4 February 1989), 299–305.)

A Critic

George Bernard Shaw
1856–1950

From *Preface on Doctors*

IT is not the fault of our doctors that the medical service of the community, as at present provided for, is a murderous absurdity. That any sane nation, having observed that you could provide for the supply of bread by giving bakers a pecuniary interest in baking for you, should go on to give a surgeon a pecuniary interest in cutting off your leg, is enough to make one despair of political humanity. But that is precisely what we have done. And the more appalling the mutilation, the more the mutilator is paid. He who corrects the ingrowing toe-nail receives a few shillings: he who cuts your inside out receives hundreds of guineas, except when he does it to a poor person for practice.

Scandalized voices murmur that these operations are necessary. They may be. It may also be necessary to hang a man or pull down a house. But we take good care not to make the hangman and the housebreaker the judges of that. If we did, no man's neck would be safe and no man's house stable. But we do make the doctor the judge, and fine him anything from sixpence to several hundred guineas if he decides in our favour. I cannot knock my shins severely without forcing on some surgeon the difficult question, 'Could I not make a better use of a pocketful of guineas than this man is making of his leg? Could he not write as well—or even better—on one leg than on two? And the guineas would make all the difference in the world to me just now. My wife—my pretty ones—the leg may mortify—it is always safer to operate—he will be well in a fortnight—artificial legs are now so well made that they are really better than natural ones—evolution is towards motors and leglessness, &c, &c, &c.'

Now there is no calculation that an engineer can make as to the behaviour of a girder under a strain, or an astronomer as to the recurrence of a comet, more certain than the calculation that under such circumstances we shall be dismembered unnecessarily in all directions by surgeons who believe the operations to be necessary solely because they want to perform them. The process metaphorically called bleeding the rich man is performed not only metaphorically but literally everyday by surgeons who are quite as honest as most of us. After all, what harm is there in it? The surgeon need not take off the rich man's (or woman's) leg or arm: he can remove the appendix or the uvula, and leave the patient none the worse after a fortnight or so in bed, whilst the nurse, the general practitioner, the apothecary, and the surgeon will be the better.

DOUBTFUL CHARACTER BORNE BY THE MEDICAL PROFESSION

Again I hear the voices indignantly muttering old phrases about the high character of a noble profession and the honour and conscience of its members. I must reply that the medical profession has not a high character: it has an infamous character. I do not know a single thoughtful and well-informed person who does not feel that the tragedy of illness at present is that it delivers you helplessly into the hands of a profession which you deeply mistrust, because it not only advocates and practises the most revolting cruelties in the pursuit of knowledge, and justifies them on grounds which would equally justify practising the same cruelties on yourself or your children, or burning down London to test a patent fire extinguisher, but, when it has shocked the public, tries to reassure it with lies of breath-bereaving brazenness. That is the character the medical profession has got just now. It may be deserved or it may not: there it is at all events; and the doctors who have not realized this are living in a fool's paradise. As to the honour and conscience of doctors, they have as much as any other class of men, no more and no less. And what other men dare pretend to be impartial where they have a strong pecuniary interest on one side? Nobody supposes that doctors are less virtuous than judges; but a judge whose salary and reputation depended on whether the verdict was for plaintiff or defendant, prosecutor or prisoner, would be as little trusted as a general in the pay of the enemy. To offer me a doctor as my judge, and then weight his decision with a bribe of a large sum of money and a virtual guarantee that if he makes a mistake it can never be proved against him, is to go wildly beyond the ascertained strain which human nature will bear. It is simply unscientific to allege or believe that doctors do not under existing circumstances perform unnecessary operations and manufacture and prolong lucrative illnesses. The only ones who can claim to be above suspicion are those who are so much sought after that their cured patients are immediately replaced by fresh ones. And there is this curious psychological fact to be remembered: a serious illness or a death advertises the doctor exactly as a hanging advertises the barrister who defended the person hanged. Suppose, for example, a royal personage gets something wrong with his throat, or has a pain in his inside. If a doctor effects some trumpery cure with a wet compress or a peppermint lozenge nobody takes the least notice of him. But if he operates on the throat and kills the patient, or extirpates an internal organ and keeps the whole nation palpitating for days whilst the patient hovers in pain and fever between life and death, his fortune is made: every rich man who omits to call him in when the same symptoms appear in his household is held not to have done his utmost duty to the patient. The wonder is that there is a king or queen left alive in Europe.

◦⁓⁑ ⁑⁓◦

Somnambulism, Vampirism, and Suicide: The Life of Dr John Polidori

Brian Hurwitz, General Practitioner
1951–
Ruth Richardson, Historian
1951–

INTRODUCTION

JOHN WILLIAM POLIDORI, an Edinburgh trained doctor, was only 20 when he was appointed personal physician to Lord Byron. His father had opposed the arrangement because he disapproved of the poet's reputation: but since the post involved accompanying Byron on a journey across Europe, the young doctor disregarded his father's scruples. Though the young Polidori's enthusiasm for the trip was soon to fade, no one could have predicted its eventual outcome: a welter of misunderstanding concerning the doctor's authorship of a celebrated gothic novel in which his lordship appeared as a vampire.

Then at the height of his literary fame, Lord Byron had become engulfed in scandal as a result of the break-up of his marriage and an incestuous relationship with his half-sister. In the spring of 1816, he had resolved to flee Britain for the Continent, leaving gossip and bad debts behind. Polidori joined the entourage accompanying Byron's great carriage, a specially commissioned copy of that owned by Napoleon, which contained bedroom, library, and 'every apparatus for dining'.

Polidori's father, Gaetano, was an Italian literary figure long settled in Soho. A teacher of Italian to the nobility, he also translated Italian poets into English, and Milton and Shakespeare into his native tongue. Of his English wife little is known. John, their eldest son, had been born in 1795 and had been sent to Ampleforth School, before studying medicine at Edinburgh during the years 1811–15.

MD THESIS: SOMNAMBULISM

Prior to his journey with Byron, the young Polidori's noteworthy written accomplishment was his MD thesis. Written in Latin, its style was conventional and derivative. Its subject, however, was unusual, for it concerned somnambulism. The epigraph chosen for its title-page was from the sleepwalking scene in Macbeth: '*A great perturbation in nature! to receive at once the benefit of sleep, and do the effects of watching.*' Polidori followed previous authorities in his discussion of the condition. Using two case histories, one of which had been communicated by a medical uncle to the Royal College of Physicians, he attempted to account for the peculiarities of sensory awareness revealed by experiments on sleepwalkers. Polidori's orientation was empirical and materialist, but he acknowledged during discussion that contemporary knowledge fell far short of explaining the phenomenon. As for treatment, Polidori followed the recommendations of de Sauvages, including the use of cold baths, flagellation, and even electricity to arouse the sleeper.

By Polidori's own account, the thesis was well received, and he passed his examination with flying colours. The experience of writing may have kindled a desire to pursue a literary career, rather than to practise as a doctor, for he soon published a pamphlet against the use of capital punishment 'for every petty offence'. Being socially well connected, his introduction to Lord Byron was facilitated by an eminent medical man of the day. Perhaps accurately, he was soon judged an 'odd dog' by Byron's best friend, Hobhouse.

TRAVELS WITH LORD BYRON

Within a week of leaving London, Polidori wrote to his favourite sister, Frances, that he was 'very pleased with Lord Byron. I am with him on the footing of an equal—everything alike.' Possibly the initial politeness of *noblesse oblige* was mistaken by the younger man as a sign of equality, which subsequently caused difficulties.

Polidori kept a diary of the trip in the belief that a fee of £500 would be forthcoming from Byron's publisher, John Murray. An edited transcript survives from which it seems not surprising that the fee never materialized. Polidori had apparently failed to appreciate the literary product Murray had in mind. Polidori is the focus of attention rather than his famous employer. Little sense of Byron's personality or preoccupations emerges: the notorious poet's energy, wit, dress, and personal foibles, all of which would have had great appeal to the book-buying public of the day, go unrecorded. Instead, the journal chronicles the well-known topography of the journey, Polidori's personal purchases and his own reactions to architecture, landscape, and local inhabitants. It reveals a rather immature and self-regarding author, entirely preoccupied with his own literary ambitions, apparently quite unaware of the literary and historical value of what he was witnessing. Polidori's biographer, D. L. Macdonald, captures the document's eccentricity; rather than being an 'account of somebody's travels with Byron', it is 'an account of Polidori's travels with somebody'.

The party left London towards the end of April 1816, but was held up in Dover for a few days due to bad weather in the Channel. Polidori lost no time in presenting his own literary efforts to the noble poet. He had brought along the manuscript, now unfortunately lost, of a play entitled *Cajetan*. Much to his chagrin, the hilarity of its critical reception by Byron set the tone for their relationship for the rest of the tour. 'Having delivered my play into their hands', Polidori confided to his diary,

> I had to hear it laughed at. . . . One of the party, however—to smoothe, I suppose, my ruffled spirits—took up my play, and apparently read part with great attention, drawing applause from those who before had laughed. He read on with such attention that others declared he had never been so attentive before.

From Ostend the Napoleonic carriage made its way across Europe to Geneva, where it arrived in late May, after a month's tour which had taken in the battlefield of Waterloo and the crags and castles of the Rhine. Mary Wollstonecraft Godwin (later Mary Shelley) and the poet Percy Bysshe Shelley had already arrived with their young son. They were accompanied by Mary's step-sister, Claire Clairmont, already pregnant by Byron, and endeavouring to prolong the affair.

TALES OF MEDICINE AND IMAGINATION: VAMPIRISM

Polidori made himself useful in arranging accommodation on the south bank of Lake Geneva. In early June the Shelleys took a small house near the shoreline, while Byron leased the Villa Diodati, a grand mansion further up the hillside. The two poets took riding and boating expeditions together in the environs of the lake. Sometimes Polidori accompanied them, but sadly, his journal records only trivialities. The doctor also spent time with Mary Shelley. They boated on the lake and read the Italian poet Tasso together. It seems likely that their discussions ranged widely, perhaps including topics such as Polidori's thesis, which he had brought along with him, and his experience as a medical student in Edinburgh at a time when copious bloodletting was customary and bodysnatching was rife. He took the young William Shelley for innoculation against smallpox and received a gold chain and seal from the child's grateful parents. On one memorable occasion, Polidori had call to administer ether to Shelley himself during a hallucinatory panic attack.

Bad weather that June had significant literary repercussions. The Villa Diodati had past associations with the poet Milton, and the setting seemed propitious for literary inspiration. With encouragement from Byron, Polidori began another play, but all agreed it was 'worth nothing'. Confined to the villa by incessant rain and electrical storms, the Shelleys often stayed overnight, and the late nights allowed long periods of talk and imaginative exchange. Mary Shelley recalled:

> Many and long were the conversations between Lord Byron and Shelley, to which I was a devout but nearly silent listener. During one of these, various philosophical doctrines were discussed, and among others the nature of the principle of life, and whether there was any probability of its ever being discovered and communicated. They talked of the experiments of Dr [Erasmus] Darwin . . . who preserved a piece of vermicelli in a glass case, till by some extraordinary means it began to move with voluntary motion.

'THE GHOST STORIES ARE BEGUN'

The literary catalyst proved to be a reading of *Fantasmagoriana, or Tales of the Dead*, a collection of German gothic stories which had recently been published in English. The opening tale featured a circle of friends whose custom it was to expect from each member 'a story of ghosts, or something of a similar nature'. The tales excited 'a playful desire of imitation', and on Lord Byron's suggestion, the friends at the Villa Diodati each agreed to attempt the creation of a gothic tale of terror.

> 'There were four of us,' Mary Shelley remembered later. 'The noble author began a tale, a fragment of which he printed at the end of his poem of Mazeppa. Shelley, more apt to embody ideas and sentiments in . . . melodious verse, than to invent the machinery of a story, commenced one founded upon the early experiences of his life. Poor Polidori had some terrible idea about a skull-headed lady . . . I busied myself *to*

think of a story to rival those which had excited us to this task. . . . I saw—with shut eyes, but acute mental vision—I saw the pale student of unhallowed arts kneeling beside the thing he had put together. I saw the hideous phantasm of a man stretched out, and then, on the working of some powerful engine, show signs of life, and stir . . .'

The two poets soon gave up the attempt to write in prose and went off into the Alps where they 'lost . . . all memory of their ghostly visions', but the curious chemistry of the Villa Diodati gave rise to two archetypal literary monsters. Mary Shelley conceived the story of *Frankenstein*, and Polidori was inspired by Byron's piece to write *The Vampyre*.

A BLOOD-LETTING TRADITION

Present-day conceptions of vampirism are largely the result of cinematic versions of *Dracula*. They derive from Bram Stoker's novel of 1897, whose vampire Count was influenced by the aristocratic original in Polidori's own vampire tale, now little known:

One Christmas a gentleman, Aubrey, meets Lord Ruthven, a nobleman in embarrassed financial circumstances. Although he is aware that others of his acquaintance had met a bad end, Aubrey is captivated and agrees to accompany Ruthven on a European tour. Rumours of licentious activities reach Aubrey's only sister, who writes from England to implore her brother's return. Instead he parts from Ruthven and travels on alone to Greece, where he falls in love.

Ignoring warnings about vampires in the locality, Aubrey takes a ride through a forest, and is attacked. When his assailant flees, the body of Aubrey's sweetheart is found nearby, drained of blood. Soon afterwards, Aubrey is seized with fever and Ruthven, newly arrived in Athens, nurses him back to health. Once again, they travel on together but are attacked by robbers, and Ruthven is shot. On his deathbed, Ruthven extracts a solemn vow from Aubrey that he shall keep Ruthven's crimes and death a secret.

On his return to London, Aubrey finds himself haunted by Ruthven's words: 'remember your oath', and goes mad. In a lucid interval he is able to congratulate his sister on her forthcoming marriage, but reacts with horror to the news that the groom is none other than Ruthven himself. His terror is mistaken for insanity. During a struggle to prevent the wedding. Aubrey bursts a blood vessel and is conveyed to his deathbed, where he reveals all before expiring at midnight. Too late—Ruthven had vanished, and Aubrey's sister had 'glutted the thirst of a VAMPYRE!'

A FRIGHTFUL PHLEBOTOMIST

The existence of Eastern European vampire lore had long been known in Britain, and the subject had recently emerged in poetry. Polidori's story, however, marked its first appearance in British prose fiction. The tale gained added power because his character, Ruthven, served to transform the hitherto shadowy ghoulish vampire figure of foreign folklore into a very English version of the dangerous gothic villain, circulating as a fine lord in high society.

Moreover, certain characteristics discernably linked Polidori's villain with Lord Byron. The villain's name, Ruthven, alluded to a bestselling sensational novel which had recently been published by Lady Caroline Lamb—another of the poet's discarded lovers—in which Byron had been only thinly disguised under the same name. Polidori, on the other hand, clearly identified himself with Aubrey, the handsome and gentle hero/victim. The bond between the hero and his sister reflects Polidori's close relationship to his own sister, Frances, and the family opposition he had experienced with regard to his own journey resurfaces in the tale. The book's central dilemma, which concerns the status of an honourable vow made to a dishonourable person, may reflect Polidori's own situation quite closely. He had observed Byron's sexual peccadilloes on the journey to Geneva; once there, he had been obliged to comply in Byron's avoidance of the pregnant Miss Clairmont.

Further parallels may be seen in the fact that Polidori and Byron separated after leaving Geneva, each travelling on alone. 'His remaining with me', Byron wrote later, 'was out of the question.' Thereafter each heard news of the other through the publisher, Murray, who later solicited from Byron a 'delicate' refusal of a play Polidori had sent in the hope of publication. Byron accordingly obliged:

> Dear Doctor—I have read your play
> Which is a good one in its way
> Purges the eyes & moves the bowels
> And drenches handkerchiefs like towels
> With tears that in a flux of Grief
> Afford hysterical relief
> To shatter'd nerves & quickened pulses
> Which your catastrophe convulses.
> Your dialogue is apt & smart
> The play's concoction full of art—
> Your hero raves—your heroine cries
> All stab—& every body dies:
> In short your tragedy would be
> The very thing to hear & see—
> And for a piece of publication
> If I decline on this occasion
> It is not that I am not sensible
> To merits in themselves ostensible

> But—and I grieve to speak it—plays
> Are drugs—mere drugs, Sir, nowadays . . .
> And so with endless truth and hurry
> Dear Doctor—I am yours
>
> John Murray.

Undaunted, Polidori continued writing after his return to England, where he set up in practice in Norwich in 1817. Paying patients were slow to materialize, and a dispensary he established for the poor was a net drain on his resources. Although Polidori tried to cut a figure among those he aspired to receive as clients, the costs proved beyond his means and he fell into debt. From a comfortable distance, Byron quipped: 'I fear the doctor's skill at Norwich will never salt the doctor's porridge' . . . and so it proved.

Polidori was at last persuaded to return to the family home at 38 Great Pulteney Street, Soho, and at this stage seems to have given up all hope of success in medicine. He began to study for the bar, and in an attempt to clear his debts published a number of pamphlets, articles, and poems. He also attempted to publish parts of his old diary, but Murray declined to take it. Polidori could easily have made money by composing a salacious memoir of the Geneva trip, but perhaps the idea did not occur to him, or for reasons of honour, or his own literary and social ambitions, he did not do so. His plans took another form. At that time, 1818–19, Polidori's former companions at the Villa Diodati had each gained considerable literary notoriety: Byron with his hilarious and licentious *Don Juan*; Shelley with his *Mask of Anarchy*, a violent attack on the government of the day; and Mary Shelley with *Frankenstein*. It was perhaps natural that Polidori should aspire to similar success.

The full story of the publication of Polidori's *Vampyre* will probably never be known. It appeared as 'a Tale by Lord Byron' in the *New Monthly Magazine* on April Fool's Day 1819. This apparent literary imposture has since been untangled by Polidori's nephew William Rossetti, and his biographer, D. L. Macdonald. It appears that the publisher attributed the tale to Byron either through a misunderstanding or, more likely, to ensure large sales. Polidori immediately publicized his own authorship of the story, stating that only the 'groundwork' had been the poet's. Despite Byron's repudiation of the piece, the association with him made the story a runaway success. Five editions were published in its first year, and the tale went on to be used as the basis for melodramas and operas. *The Vampyre* was widely acclaimed, particularly on the Continent, where Goethe even declared it to be Byron's best work.

SUICIDE: A MELANCHOLY EVENT

Polidori had sold his manuscript for a fee rather than a royalty, and his tale was published before the days of copyright, so even though it became a bestseller, the author himself earned very little from it. When his other literary ventures failed, the young man turned to gambling, which only aggravated his financial distress. One morning in August 1821 he was found dying in the family house at Great Pulteney Street.

Thomas Copeland, the medical man called urgently to attend him, applied a stomach pump, but Polidori died within minutes. At the inquest, the coroner's jury recorded a verdict of 'died by the visitation of God', which implied death by natural causes without stating an exact diagnosis. No post-mortem had been performed. Five members of the twelve-man jury came from Great Pulteney Street itself, and the remainder from its close vicinity. Their deliberations were made in the Polidori family house. It would not have been an unknown occurrence at that time if consideration for a family's grief and honour had led neighbours to avoid inflicting the disgrace of a verdict of *felo de se* or suicide.

The real cause of death remains open to contention. It is said to have been common knowledge within the Polidori family that he had taken prussic acid. The likelihood of suicide also occurred to others. Byron commented on hearing the news: 'Poor Polidori is gone. When he was my physician he was always talking of prussic acid, oil of amber, blowing into veins, suffocating by charcoal, and compounding poisons.'

His father, on going through his son's belongings, was sadly impressed by the volume of his writings: 'He has left such a quantity of manuscripts, literary, philosophical, and poetical, that it seems impossible that a young man who lived only twenty-five years could have thought and written so much.'

No stone survives today to mark Polidori's grave in St Pancras old burial ground, and no plaque marks the family home which still stands. Though Polidori himself is now almost forgotten, the spirit of that summer at the Villa Diodati resonates on into our own times. The young doctor may well have influenced the creation of Mary Shelley's *Frankenstein*, while in the popular imagination the progeny of his own *Vampyre* continue to feed on their unsuspecting prey.

(The fully referenced version can be found in the *Proceedings of the Royal College of Physicians, Edinburgh*, **21** (1991), 458–66.)

❦4❧

Nurses and Patients

NURSES are linked in the contemporary consciousness with the squeaky-clean conditions of the modern hospital. But of course modern nursing has its origins in the appalling conditions of field hospitals, which are described by Florence Nightingale. It is also easy to forget about the many contexts in which the modern nurse works, and a more specialized work would need to include material on midwives and the male nurse. But I have included a few important people from porters to chaplains whose work is often ignored.

Patients, of course, are at the centre of health care, but patients are closely associated with ambulances, hospitals, visitors, chaplains, and many other aspects of health care. There is one other side to health care which nowadays threatens to engulf all the others—management. The piece by an anonymous writer to the Lancet in the 1960s is prophetic of what has now come about.

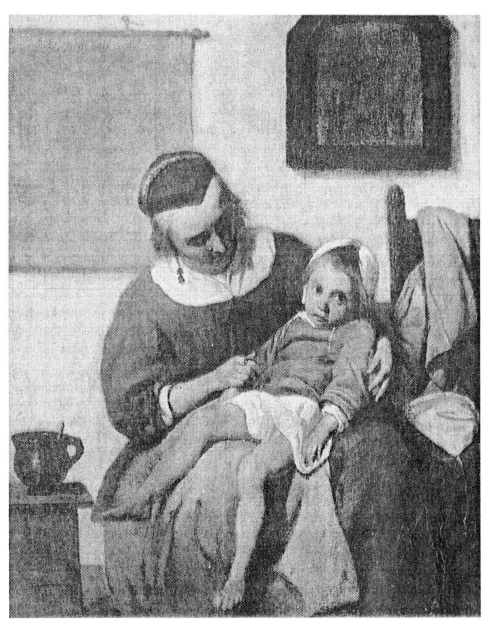

The Sick Child (c. 1665). *Gabriel Metsu.*
This child is obviously being well looked after. Nursing had to wait some hundreds of years before it became a profession, but in the compassionate but observant posture of the adult woman one can see the qualities of the modern nurse.

Nurses

John Betjeman
1906–1984

Death in Leamington

SHE died in the upstairs bedroom
  By the light of the evening star
That shone through the plate glass window
  From over Leamington Spa.

Beside her the lonely crochet
  Lay patiently and unstirred,
But the fingers that would have worked it
  Were dead as the spoken word.

And Nurse came in with the tea-things
  Breast high 'mid the stands and chairs—
But Nurse was alone with her own little soul,
  And the things were alone with theirs.

She bolted the big round window,
  She let the blinds unroll,
She set a match to the mantle,
  She covered the fire with coal.

And "Tea!" she said in a tiny voice
  "Wake up! It's nearly *five*."
Oh! Chintzy, chintzy cheeriness,
  Half dead and half alive!

Do you know that the stucco is peeling?
　　Do you know that the heart will stop?
From those yellow Italianate archcs
　　Do you hear the plaster drop?

Nurse looked at the silent bedstead,
　　At the gray, decaying face,
As the calm of a Leamington evening
　　Drifted into the place.

She moved the table of bottles
　　Away from the bed to the wall;
And tiptoeing gently over the stairs
　　Turned down the gas in the hall.

Florence Nightingale
1820–1910

The State of the Wards

A LETTER from Miss Nightingale herself to her friend of Harley Street, Dr Bowman, the ophthalmic surgeon, gives a lively account of some of her difficulties, and a vivid picture of the horrors amid which her work was done (Nov. 14):

'*I came out, Ma'am, prepared to submit to everything, to be put upon in every way. But there are some things, Ma'am, one can't submit to. There is the Caps, Ma'am, that suits one face, and some that suits another. And if I'd known, Ma'am, about the Caps, great as was my desire to come out to nurse at Scutari, I wouldn't have come, Ma'am.*' —*Speech of Mrs Lawfield.*—Time must be at a discount with the man who can adjust the balance of such an important question as the above, and I for one have none: as you will easily suppose when I tell you that on Thursday last we had 1715 sick and wounded in this Hospital (among whom 120 Cholera Patients), and 650 severely wounded in the other Building called the General Hospital, of which we also have charge, when a message came to me to prepare for 510 wounded on our side of the Hospital who were arriving from the dreadful affair of the 5th November from Balaklava, in which battle were 1,763 wounded and 442 killed, besides 96 officers wounded and 38 killed. I always expected to end my Days as Hospital Matron, but I never expected to be Barrack Mistress. We had but half an hour's notice before they began landing the wounded. Between 1 and 9 o'clock we had the mattresses stuffed, sewn up, laid down—alas! only upon matting on the floor—the men washed and put to bed, and all their wounds dressed. I wish I had time. I would write you a letter dear to a surgeon's heart. I am as good as a *Medical Times*! But oh! you Gentlemen of England who sit at Home in all the well-earned satisfaction of your successful cases, can have little Idea from reading the newspapers of the Horror and Misery (in a Military Hospital) of operating upon these dying, exhausted men. A London Hospital is a Garden of Flowers to it.

We have had such a Sea in the Bosphorus, and the Turks, the very men for whom we are fighting, carry in our Wounded so cruelly, that they arrive in a state of Agony. One amputated Stump died 2 hours after we received him, one compound Fracture just as we were getting him into Bed—in all, twenty-four cases died on the day of landing. The Dysentery Cases have died at the rate of one in two. Then the day of operations which follows. . . .

We are very lucky in our Medical Heads. Two of them are brutes, and four are angels—for this is a work which makes either angels or devils of men and of women too. As for the assistants, they are all Cubs, and will, while a man is breathing his last breath under the knife, lament the 'annoyance of being called up from their dinners by such a fresh influx of wounded'! But unlicked Cubs grow up into good old Bears, tho' I don't know how; for certain it is the old Bears are good. We have now *four miles* of Beds, and not eighteen inches apart.

We have our Quarters in one Tower of the Barrack, and all this fresh influx has been laid down between us and the Main Guard, in two Corridors, with a line of Beds down each side, just room for one person to pass between, and four wards. Yet in the midst of this appalling Horror (we are steeped up to our necks in blood) there is good, and I can truly say, like St Peter, 'It is good for us to be here'— though I doubt whether if St Peter had been here, he would have said so. As I went my night-rounds among the newly wounded that first night, there was not one murmur, not one groan, the strictest discipline—the most absolute silence and quiet prevailed—only the steps of the Sentry—and I heard one man say, 'I was dreaming of my friends at Home,' and another said, 'I was thinking of them.' These poor fellows bear pain and mutilation with an unshrinking heroism which is really superhuman, and die, or are cut up without a complaint.

The wounded are now lying up to our very door, and we are landing 540 more from the *Andes*. I take rank in the Army as Brigadier General, because 40 British females, whom I have with me, are more difficult to manage than 4,000 men. Let no lady come out here who is not used to fatigue and privation. . . . Every ten minutes an Orderly runs, and we have to go and cram lint into the wound till a Surgeon can be sent for, and stop the Bleeding as well as we can. In all our corridor, I think we have not an average of three Limbs per man. And there are two Ships more 'loading' at the Crimea with wounded—(this is our Phraseology). Then come the operations, and a melancholy, not an encouraging List is this. They are all performed in the wards—no time to move them; one poor fellow exhausted with haemorrhage, has his leg amputated as a last hope, and dies ten minutes after the Surgeon has left him. Almost before the breath has left his body it is sewn up in its blanket, and carried away and buried the same day. We have no room for Corpses in the Wards. The Surgeons pass on to the next, an excision of the shoulder-joint, beautifully performed and going on well. Ball lodged just in the head of the joint and fracture starred all round. The next poor fellow has two Stumps for arms, and the next has lost an arm and a leg. As for the Balls they go in where they like and come out where they like and do as much harm as they can in passing. That is the only rule they have. . . .

I am getting a Screen now for the amputations, for when one poor fellow, who is to be amputated tomorrow sees his comrade today die under the knife, it makes impression and diminishes his chance. But, anyway, among these exhausted Frames, the mortality of the operations is frightful. We have Erysipelas, fever, and gangrene, and the Russian wounded are the worst.

We are getting on nicely though in many ways. They were so glad to see us. The Senior Chaplain is a sensible man, which is a remarkable Providence. . . . If you ever see Mr Whitfield, the House Apothecary of St Thomas's, will you tell him that the nurse he sent me, Mrs Roberts, is worth her weight in gold. . . . Mrs Drake is a Treasure. The four others are not fit to take care of themselves, but they may do better by and by if I can convince them of the absolute necessity of discipline. We hear there was another engagement on the 8th and more wounded, who are coming down to us. This is only the beginning of things.

Wilfred Owen
1893–1918

Conscious

HIS fingers wake, and flutter; up the bed.
His eyes come open with a pull of will,
Helped by the yellow mayflowers by his head.
The blind-cord drawls across the window-sill . . .
What a smooth floor the ward has! What a rug!
Who is that talking somewhere out of sight?
Three flies are creeping round the shiny jug . . .
'Nurse! Doctor!'—'Yes; all right, all right.'

But sudden evening blurs and fogs the air.
There seems no time to want a drink of water,
Nurse looks so far away. And here and there
Music and roses burst through crimson slaughter.
He can't remember where he saw blue sky . . .
The trench is narrower. Cold, he's cold; yet hot—
And there's no light to see the voices by . . .
There is no time to ask . . . he knows not what.

Miss G. M. Mitchell
(dates unknown)

The Nurse

HERE in the long white ward I stand,
  Pausing a little breathless space,
Touching a restless fevered hand,
  mouthing comfort's commonplace—

Long enough pause to feel the cold
  Fingers of fear about my heart;
Just for the moment, uncontrolled,
  All the pent tears of pity start.

While here I strive, as best I may,
   Strangers' long hours of pain to ease,
Dumbly I question—Far away
   Lies my beloved even as these?

(1916)

Charles Dickens
1812–1870
From *Martin Chuzzlewit*
[*Mrs Gamp*]

'WHY, highty tighty, sir!' cried Mrs Gamp, 'is these your manners? You want a pitcher of cold water throw'd over you to bring you round; that's my belief; and if you was under Betsey Prig you'd have it, too, I do assure you, Mr Chuffey. Spanish Flies is the only thing to draw this nonsense out of you, and if anybody wanted to do you a kindness, they'd clap a blister of 'em on your head, and put a mustard poultige on your back. Who's dead, indeed! It wouldn't be no grievous loss if someone was, I think!'

'He's quiet now, Mrs Gamp,' said Merry. 'Don't disturb him.'

'Oh, bother the old wictim, Mrs Chuzzlewit,' replied that zealous lady. 'I ain't no patience with him. You give him his own way too much by half. A worritin' wexagious creetur!'

No doubt with the view of carrying out the precepts she enforced, and 'bothering the old wictim' in practice as well as in theory, Mrs Gamp took him by the collar of his coat, and gave him some dozen or two of hearty shakes backward and forward in his chair; that exercise being considered by the disciples of the Prig school of nursing (who are very numerous among professional ladies) as exceedingly conducive to repose, and highly beneficial to the performance of the nervous functions. Its effect in this instance was to render the patient so giddy and addle-headed, that he could say nothing more; which Mrs Gamp regarded as the triumph of her art.

'There!' she said, loosening the old man's cravat, in consequence of his being rather black in the face, after this scientific treatment. 'Now, I hope, you're easy in your mind. If you should turn at all faint we can soon revive you, sir, I promige you. Bite a person's thumbs, or turn their fingers the wrong way,' said Mrs Gamp, smiling with the consciousness of at once imparting pleasure and instruction to her auditors, 'and they comes to, wonderful, Lord bless you!'

Janice Galloway
1956–

From *The Trick is to Keep Breathing*

The Health Visitor

BY twenty past I'm running along the twisty road between the houses to the shop for biscuits. She likes biscuits. I get different ones each time hoping they are something else she will enjoy. I can't choose in a hurry. I can't be trusted with custard creams so deliberately don't get them. Chocolate digestives are too expensive. I wait for too long in the queue while a confused little kid tries to bargain for his father's cigarettes with the wrong money, so I have to run back clutching fig rolls and iced coffees and nearly drop the milk. I get flustered at these times, but I know I'll manage if I try harder. These visits are good for me. Dr Stead sends this woman out of love. He insisted.

I said, I'm no use with strangers.

He said, But this is different. Health Visitors are trained to cope with that. He said she would know what to do; she would find me out and let me talk. *Make me talk.*

HAH

I'm putting on the kettle, still catching my breath when she comes in without knocking and frightens me. What if I had been saying things about her out loud? I tell her to sit in the livingroom so I can have time to think.

Tray

       jug

              sweeteners

                    plates

                          cups and saucers

                                another spoon

                                    christ

the biscuits
the biscuits

I burst the wrap soundlessly and make a tasteful arrangement. I polish her teaspoon on my cardigan band. No teapot. I make it in the cup, using the same bag twice, and take it through as though I've really made it in a pot and just poured it out. Some people are sniffy about tea-bags. It sloshes when I reach to push my hair back from falling in my eyes and I suddenly notice I am still wearing my slippers dammit.
Never mind. She smiles and says

This is to make out the tea is a surprise though it isn't. She does it every time. We sit opposite each other because that's the way the chairs are. The chairs cough dust from under their sheets as she crosses her legs, thinking her way into the part. By the time she's ready to start I'm grinding my teeth back into the gum.

HEALTH VISITOR So, how are you/ how's life/ what's been happening/
anything interesting to tell me/ what's new?
PATIENT   Oh, fine/ nothing to speak of.

I stir the tea repeatedly. She picks a piece of fluff off her skirt.

HEALTH VISITOR Work. How are things at work? Coping?
PATIENT   Fine. [Pause] I have trouble getting in on time, but getting
better.

I throw her a little difficulty every so often so she feels I'm telling her the truth. I figure this will get rid of her quicker.

HEALTH VISITOR [Intensifying] But what about the day-to-day? How are you
coping?
PATIENT   OK. [Brave smile] I manage.
HEALTH VISITOR The house is looking fine.
PATIENT   Thank-you. I do my best.

This is overdone. She flicks her eyes up to see and I lower mine. She reaches for a biscuit.

HEALTH VISITOR These look nice. I like a biscuit with a cup of tea.

We improvise about the biscuits for a while, her hat sliding back as she chews. She doesn't like the tea. Maybe she eats so many biscuits just to get rid of the taste.

HEALTH VISITOR Aren't you having one? They're very good.
PATIENT No, thanks. Maybe later. Having lunch soon.

She goes on munching, knowing I don't want her to be here/ that I do want her to be here but I can't talk to her.

This is the fourth time we have played this fucking game.

The first time was worst. I went through the tea ceremony for five minutes then tried to get the thing opened up.

What are you supposed to come here for? I said. She just looked.
What's it for? What are we supposed to talk about?
She said, I'm here to help you. To help you try to get better. I'm here to listen.
But I don't know you from a hole in the wall. I can't do it.
She said, You can tell me anything you like. I assure you it goes no further and I've heard it all before.

I could hear my own breathing. I knew Dr Stead was doing his best for me and that was why she was here. I had to try. It was reasonable. I swallowed hard. I can't remember what I said now. Whatever it was, I was in mid-flow, keeping my eyes low because I couldn't look her in the eye. When I finished, nothing happened. I looked up.

She was dunking a gingernut. I watched her hand rocking back and forth, getting the saturation just right. At the crucial moment, she flipped the biscuit to her mouth, sucking off the soaked part, her tongue worming out for a dribble of tea. It missed. The dribble ran down to her chin and she coughed, giggling. And I had forgotten what I had to say. I knew if I opened my mouth something terrible would dribble out like tea, gush down the front of my shirt, over her shoes and cover the carpet like
like
like

She sucked her teeth and leaned closer, whispering.

She knew how I felt. Did I think doctor hadn't given her case notes? She knew all about my problems. Did I want her to tell me a true story? Her

niece had an accident on her bike once. And she thought, what'll happen if
Angela dies? what'll happen? But she prayed to God and the family rallied
round and they saw her through to the other side. That's what I had to
remember. She knew how I felt; she knew exactly how I felt.

She keeps coming anyway. I make tea and fetch biscuits and we forget all
about that first little hiccup. This time she eats only the coffee biscuits so I
make a mental note. No more fig rolls. The way I'm coiled is getting
uncomfortable. One foot has gone to sleep and my tea is coated. I put it
down on the rug and straighten up.

HEALTH VISITOR [Alert to the change] Nothing else to tell me, then?
PATIENT   No. Nothing special.

She looks blank and vaguely disappointed. I am not trying.

PATIENT   I have a friend visiting tonight. That's all.
HEALTH VISITOR Anyone special? Going out?
PATIENT   Just the pub, have a few drinks, that kind of thing.
HEALTH VISITOR Lucky girl. I can't remember the last time someone took me
                     out. Lucky.

She smiles and stands up but guilt is spoiling the relief. I get more guilty as
she waddles towards the door, tumbling crumbs from the folds of blue coat,
fastening up one top button, ready for outside. My temples thunder as she
touches the door and something buzzes in my ear.

You Always Expect Too Much.

The exhaust rattles till she curves out of sight, struggling against her bulk
and the need to turn the wheel.

I rub out the creases on the chairs where we have been sitting then take the
crockery through and crash it into the sink. One of the red cups has a hairline
crack along the rim, fine but deep enough to cut if it wanted. I throw the cup
in the bin in case the person it cuts is not me. I lift the biscuits still on the
plate and crush them between my hands into the bin. The opened packets
follow. They only go soft. The wrappers crackle with life in the recesses of
the liner so I let the lid drop fast and turn on the taps to drown it out. They
run too hard and soak the front of my shirt. There isn't time to change. I get
my coat and run like hell for the stop.

Ambulances and Hospitals

Philip Larkin
1922–1985

Ambulances

CLOSED like confessionals, they thread
Loud noons of cities, giving back
None of the glances they absorb.
Light glossy grey, arms on a plaque,
They come to rest at any kerb:
All streets in time are visited.

Then children strewn on steps or road,
Or women coming from the shops
Past smells of different dinners, see
A wild white face that overtops
Red stretcher-blankets momently
As it is carried in and stowed,

And sense the solving emptiness
That lies just under all we do,
And for a second get it whole,
So permanent and blank and true.
The fastened doors recede. *Poor soul,*
They whisper at their own distress;

For borne away in deadened air
May go the sudden shut of loss
Round something nearly at an end,
And what cohered in it across
The years, the unique random blend
Of families and fashions, there

At last begin to loosen. Far
From the exchange of love to lie
Unreachable inside a room
The traffic parts to let go by
Brings closer what is left to come.
And dulls to distance all we are.

John Betjeman
1906–1984

The Cottage Hospital

AT the end of a long-walled garden
   in a red provincial town,
A brick path led to a mulberry—
   scanty grass at its feet.
I lay under blackening branches
   where the mulberry leaves hung down
Sheltering ruby fruit globes
   from a Sunday-tea-time heat.
Apple and plum espaliers
   basked upon bricks of brown;
The air was swimming with insects,
   and children played in the street.

Out of this bright intentness
   into the mulberry shade
Musca domestica (housefly)
   swung from the August light

Slap into slithery rigging
   by the waiting spider made
Which spun the lithe elastic
   till the fly was shrouded tight.
Down came the hairy talons
   and horrible poison blade
And none of the garden noticed
   that fizzing, hopeless fight.

Say in what Cottage Hospital
   whose pale green walls resound
With the tap upon polished parquet
   of inflexible nurses' feet
Shall I myself be lying
   when they range the screens around?
And say shall I groan in dying,
   as I twist the sweaty sheet?
Or gasp for breath uncrying,
   as I feel my senses drown'd
While the air is swimming with insects
   and children play in the street?

Philip Larkin
1922–1985

The Building

HIGHER than the handsomest hotel
The lucent comb shows up for miles, but see,
All round it close-ribbed streets rise and fall
Like a great sigh out of the last century.
The porters are scruffy; what keep drawing up
At the entrance are not taxis; and in the hall
As well as creepers hangs a frightening smell.

There are paperbacks, and tea at so much a cup,
Like an airport lounge, but those who tamely sit
On rows of steel chairs turning the ripped mags
Haven't come far. More like a local bus,
These outdoor clothes and half-filled shopping bags
And faces restless and resigned, although
Every few minutes comes a kind of nurse

To fetch someone away: the rest refit
Cups back to saucers, cough, or glance below
Seats for dropped gloves or cards. Humans, caught
On ground curiously neutral, homes and names
Suddenly in abeyance; some are young,
Some old, but most at that vague age that claims
The end of choice, the last of hope; and all

Here to confess that something has gone wrong.
It must be error of a serious sort,
For see how many floors it needs, how tall
It's grown by now, and how much money goes
In trying to correct it. See the time,
Half-past eleven on a working day,
And these picked out of it; see, as they climb

To their appointed levels, how their eyes
Go to each other, guessing; on the way
Someone's wheeled past, in washed-to-rags ward
   clothes:
They see him, too. They're quiet. To realize
This new thing held in common makes them quiet,
For past these doors are rooms, and rooms past those,
And more rooms yet, each one further off

And harder to return from; and who knows
Which he will see, and when? For the moment, wait,
Look down at the yard. Outside seems old enough:
Red brick, lagged pipes, and someone walking by it
Out to the car park, free. Then, past the gate,
Traffic; a locked church; short terraced streets
Where kids chalk games, and girls with hair-dos fetch

Their separates from the cleaners—O world,
Your loves, your chances, are beyond the stretch
Of any hand from here! And so, unreal,
A touching dream to which we all are lulled
But wake from separately. In it, conceits
And self-protecting ignorance congeal
To carry life, collapsing only when

Called to these corridors (for now once more
The nurse beckons—). Each gets up and goes
At last. Some will be out by lunch, or four;
Others, not knowing it, have come to join
The unseen congregations whose white rows
Lie set apart above—women, men;
Old, young; crude facets of the only coin

This place accepts. All know they are going to die.
Not yet, perhaps not here, but in the end,
And somewhere like this. That is what it means,
This clean-sliced cliff; a struggle to transcend
The thought of dying, for unless its powers
Outbuild cathedrals nothing contravenes
The coming dark, though crowds each evening try

With wasteful, weak, propitiatory flowers.

Fleur Adcock
1934–

The Soho Hospital for Women

I

STRANGE room, from this angle:
white door open before me,
strange bed, mechanical hum, white lights.
There will be stranger rooms to come.

As I almost slept I saw the deep flower opening
and leaned over into it, gratefully.
It swimmingly closed in my face. I was not ready.
It was not death, it was acceptance.

                              *

Our thin patient cat died purring,
her small triangular head tilted back,
the nurse's fingers caressing her throat,
my hand on her shrunken spine; the quick needle.

That was the second death by cancer.
The first is not for me to speak of.
It was telephone calls and brave letters
and a friend's hand bleeding under the coffin.

                              *

Doctor, I am not afraid of a word.
But neither do I wish to embrace that visitor,
to engulf it as Hine-Nui-te-Po
engulfed Maui; that would be the way of it.

And she was the winner there: her womb crushed him.
Goddesses can do these things.
But I have admitted the gloved hands and the speculum
and must part my ordinary legs to the surgeon's knife.

II

Nellie has only one breast
ample enough to make several.
Her quilted dressing-gown softens
to semi-doubtful this imbalance
and there's no starched vanity
in our abundant ward-mother:
her silvery hair's in braids, her slippers
loll, her weathered smile holds true.
When she dresses up in her black
with her glittering marcasite brooch on
to go for the weekly radium treatment
she's the bright star of the taxi-party—
whatever may be growing under her ribs.

*

Doris hardly smokes in the ward—
and hardly eats more than a dreamy spoonful—
but the corridors and bathrooms
reek of her Players Number 10,
and the drug-trolley pauses
for long minutes by her bed.
Each week for the taxi-outing
she puts on her skirt again
and has to pin the slack waistband
more tightly over her scarlet sweater.
Her face, a white shadow through smoked glass,
lets Soho display itself unregarded.

*

Third in the car is Mrs Golding
who never smiles. And why should she?

III

The senior consultant on his rounds
murmurs in so subdued a voice
to the students marshalled behind
that they gather in, forming a cell,
a cluster, a rosette around him
as he stands at the foot of my bed
going through my notes with them,
half-audibly instructive, grave.

The slight ache as I strain forward
to listen still seems imagined.

Then he turns his practised smile on me:
'How are you this morning?' 'Fine,
very well, thank you.' I smile too.
And possibly all that murmurs within me
is the slow dissolving of stitches.

IV

I am out in the supermarket choosing—
this very afternoon, this day—
picking up tomatoes, cheese, bread,

things I want and shall be using
to make myself a meal, while they
eat their stodgy suppers in bed:

Janet with her big freckled breasts,
her prim Scots voice, her one friend,
and never in hospital before,

who came in to have a few tests
and now can't see where they'll end;
and Coral in the bed by the door

who whimpered and gasped behind a screen
with nurses to and fro all night
and far too much of the day;

pallid, bewildered, nineteen.
And Mary, who will be all right
but gradually. And Alice, who may.

Whereas I stand almost intact,
giddy with freedom, not with pain.
I lift my light basket, observing

how little I need in fact;
and move to the checkout, to the rain,
to the lights and the long street curving.

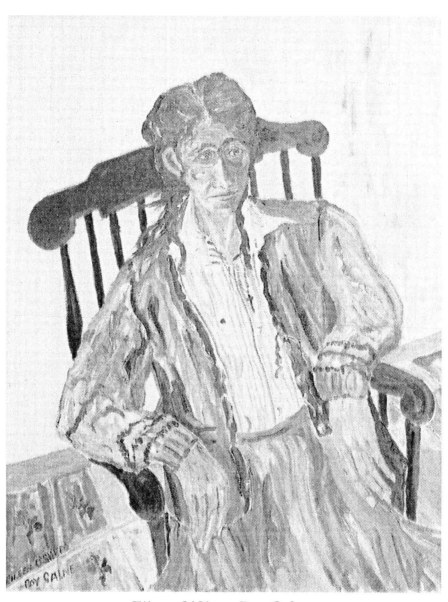

Eileen O'Shea. *Roy Calne.*
Sir Roy Calne is Professor of Surgery at Addenbrooke's Hospital, Cambridge, and a pioneer in liver transplantation. He is also a distinguished painter. In this portrait of Eileen O'Shea, who was a nurse, the three roses represent three liver transplant operations. After the portrait was painted she had a fourth, which was successful.

Patients, Visitors, and Chaplains

Elizabeth Jennings
1926–

Pain

AT my wits' end
And all resources gone, I lie here,
All of my body tense to the touch of fear,
And my mind,

Muffled now as if the nerves
Refused any longer to let thoughts form,
Is no longer a safe retreat, a tidy home,
No longer serves

My body's demands or shields
With fine words, as it once would daily,
My storehouse of dread. Now, slowly,
My heart, hand, whole body yield

To fear. Bed, ward, window begin
To lose their solidity. Faces no longer
Look kind or needed; yet I still fight the stronger
Terror—oblivion—the needle thrusts in.

D. H. Lawrence
1885–1930

Malade

THE sick grapes on the chair by the bed lie prone; at
    the window
The tassel of blind swings constantly, tapping the
    pane
As the air moves in.

The room is the hollow rind of a fruit, a gourd
Scooped out and bare, where a spider,
Folded in its legs as in a bed,
Lies on the dust, watching where there is nothing to
    see but dusky walls.

And if the day outside were mine! What is the day
But a grey cave, with great spider-cloths hanging
Low from the roof, and the wet dust falling softly
    from them
Over the wet dark rocks, the houses, and over
The spiders with white faces, that scuttle on the floor
    of the cave!

Ah, but I am ill, and it is still raining, coldly raining!

U. A. Fanthorpe
1929–

After Visiting Hours

LIKE gulls they are still calling—
I'll come again Tuesday. Our Dad
Sends his love. They diminish, are gone.
Their world has received them,

As our world confirms us. Their debris
Is tidied into vases, lockers, minds.
We become pulses; mouthpieces
Of thermometers and bowels.

The trolley's rattle dispatches
The last lover. Now we can relax
Into illness, and reliably abstracted
Nurses will straighten our sheets,

Reorganize our symptoms. Outside,
Darkness descends like an eyelid.
It rains on our nearest and dearest
In car-parks, at bus-stops.

Now the bed-bound rehearse
Their repertoire of movements,
The dressing-gowned shuffle, clutching
Their glass bodies.

Now siren voices whisper
From headphones, and vagrant
Doctors appear, wreathed in stethoscopes
Like South Sea dancers.

All's well, all's quiet as the great
Ark noses her way into the night,
Caulked, battened, blessed for her trip,
And behind, the gulls crying.

Tessa Ransford
1938–

Hospitalization

ILLNESS tossed you over the rails
of our world—
the huge hospital swallowed you
then swam away
to go through its routines with you
deep and distant.

I could no more than paddle in
that element—
but came often to watch from the shore
and scan the surface.

After a secret number of days
and hidden nights,
after fathomless hours enclosed
in the whale's belly
floating on tides of attention
and murmurs of movement,
the hospital will spit you out again
at my feet.

The sand is suddenly swept with
scuttling pebbles
sprays of scum and shells
as you come up on it.
I begin to lead you home, only
to discover
we are on a foreign shore.

Charles Lamb
1775–1834

The Convalescent

A PRETTY severe fit of indisposition which, under the name of a nervous fever, has made a prisoner of me for some weeks past, and is but slowly leaving me, has reduced me to an incapacity of reflecting upon any topic foreign to itself. Expect no healthy conclusions from me this month, reader; I can offer you only sick men's dreams.

And truly the whole state of sickness is such; for what else is it but a magnificent dream for a man to lie a-bed, and draw daylight curtains about him; and, shutting out the sun, to induce a total oblivion of all the works which are going on under it? To become insensible to all the operations of life, except the beatings of one feeble pulse?

If there be a regal solitude, it is a sick bed. How the patient lords it there; what caprices he acts without control! how king-like he sways his pillow—tumbling and tossing, and shifting, and lowering, and thumping, and flatting, and moulding it, to the ever varying requisitions of his throbbing temples.

He changes *sides* oftener than a politician. Now he lies full length, then half-length, obliquely, transversely, head and feet quite across the bed; and none accuses him of tergiversation. Within the four curtains he is absolute. They are his Mare Clausum.

How sickness enlarges the dimensions of a man's self to himself; he is his own exclusive object. Supreme selfishness is inculcated upon him as his only duty. 'Tis the Two Tables of the Law to him. He has nothing to think of but how to get well. What passes out of doors, or within them, so he hear not the jarring of them, affects him not.

A little while ago he was greatly concerned in the event of a law-suit, which was to be the making or the marring of his dearest friend. He was to be seen trudging about upon this man's errand to fifty quarters of the town at once, jogging this witness, refreshing that solicitor. The cause was to come on yesterday. He is absolutely as indifferent to the decision, as if it were a question to be tried at Pekin. Peradventure from some whispering, going on about the house, not intended for his hearing, he picks up enough to make him understand, that things went cross-grained in the Court yesterday, and his friend is ruined. But the word 'friend', and the word 'ruin', disturb him no more than so much jargon. He is not to think of anything but how to get better.

What a world of foreign cares are merged in that absorbing consideration!

He has put on his strong armour of sickness, he is wrapped in the callous hide of suffering, he keeps his sympathy, like some curious vintage, under trusty lock and key, for his own use only.

He lies pitying himself, honing and moaning to himself; he yearneth over himself; his bowels are even melted within him, to think what he suffers; he is not ashamed to weep over himself.

He is for ever plotting how to do some good to himself; studying little stratagems and artificial alleviations.

He makes the most of himself; dividing himself, by an allowable fiction, into as many distinct individuals, as he hath sore and sorrowing members. Sometimes he meditates—as of a thing apart from him—upon his poor aching head, and that dull pain which, dozing or waking, lay in it all the past night like a log, or palpable substance of pain, not to be removed without opening the very skull, as it seemed, to take it thence. Or he pities his long, clammy, attenuated fingers. He compassionates himself all over; and his bed is a very discipline of humanity, and tender heart.

He is his own sympathiser; and instinctively feels that none can so well perform that office for him. He cares for few spectators to his tragedy. Only that punctual face of the old nurse pleases him, that announces his broths, and his cordials. He likes it because it is so unmoved, and because he can pour forth his feverish ejaculations before it as unreservedly as to his bed-post.

To the world's business he is dead. He understands not what the callings and occupations of mortals are; only he has a glimmering conceit of some such thing, when the doctor makes his daily call: and even in the lines on that busy face he reads no multiplicity of patients, but solely conceives of himself as *the sick man.* To what other uneasy couch the good man is hastening, when he slips out of his chamber, folding up his thin douceur so carefully for fear of rustling—is no speculation which he can at present entertain. He thinks only of the regular return of the same phenomenon at the same hour tomorrow.

Household rumours touch him not. Some faint murmur, indicative of life going on within the house, soothes him, while he knows not distinctly what it is. He is not to know anything, not to think of anything. Servants gliding up or down the distant staircase, treading as upon velvet, gently keep his ear awake, so long as he troubles not himself further than with some feeble guess at their errands. Exacter knowledge would be a burthen to him: he can just endure the pressure of conjecture. He opens his eye faintly at the dull stroke of the muffled knocker, and closes it again without asking 'Who was it?' He is flattered by a general notion that enquiries are making after him, but he cares not to know the name of the enquirer. In the general stillness, and awful hush of the house, he lies in state, and feels his sovereignty.

To be sick is to enjoy monarchial prerogatives. Compare the silent tread, and quiet ministry, almost by the eye only, with which he is served—with the careless demeanour, the unceremonious goings in and out (slapping of doors, or leaving them open) of the very same attendants, when he is getting a little better—and you will confess, that from the bed of sickness (throne let me rather call it) to the elbow chair of convalescence, is a fall from dignity, amounting to a deposition.

How convalescence shrinks a man back to his pristine stature! Where is now the space, which he occupied so lately, in his own, in the family's eye?

The scene of his regalities, his sick room, which was his presence chamber, where he lay and acted his despotic fancies—how is it reduced to a common bed-room! The trimness of the very bed has something petty and unmeaning about it. It is *made* everyday. How unlike to that wavy many-furrowed, oceanic surface, which it presented so short a time since, when to *make* it was a service not to be thought of at oftener than three or four day revolutions, when the patient was with pain and grief to be lifted for a little while out of it, to submit to the encroachment of unwelcome neatness, and decencies which his shaken frame deprecated; then to be lifted into it again, for another three or four days' respite, to flounder it out of shape again, while every fresh furrow was a historical record of some shifting posture, some uneasy turning, some seeking for a little ease; and the shrunken skin scarce told a truer story than the crumpled coverlid.

Hushed are those mysterious sights—those groans—so much more awful, while we knew not from what caverns of vast hidden suffering they proceeded. The Lernean pangs are quenched. The riddle of sickness is solved; and Philoctetes is become an ordinary personage.

Perhaps some relic of the sick man's dream of greatness survives in the still lingering visitations of the medical attendant. But how is he too changed with everything else! Can this be he—this man of news—of chat—of anecdote—of everything but physic—can this be he, who so lately came between the patient and his cruel enemy, as on some solemn embassy from Nature, erecting herself into a high mediating party?—Pshaw! 'tis some old woman.

Farewell with him all that made sickness pompous—the spell that hushed the household—the desert-like stillness, felt throughout its inmost chambers—the mute attendance—the inquiry by looks—the still softer delicacies of self-attention

—the sole and single eye of distemper alonely fixed upon itself—world-thoughts excluded—the man a world unto himself—his own theatre—

What a speck is he dwindled into!

In this flat swamp of convalescence, left by the ebb of sickness, yet far enough from the terra firma of established health, your note, dear Editor, reached me, requesting—an article. In Articulo Mortis, thought I; but it is something hard—and the quibble, wretched as it was, relieved me. The summons, unseasonable as it appeared, seemed to link me on again to the petty businesses of life, which I had lost sight of; a gentle call to activity, however trivial; a wholesome weaning from that preposterous dream of self-absorption—the puffy state of sickness—in which I confess to have lain so long, insensible to the magazines and monarchies, of the world alike; to its laws and to its literature. The hypochondriac flatus is subsiding; the acres, which in imagination I had spread over—for the sick man swells in the sole contemplation of his single sufferings, till he becomes a Tityus to himself—are wasting to a span; and for the giant of self-importance, which I was so lately, you have me once again in my natural pretensions—the lean and meagre figure of your insignificant Essayist.

Joseph Heller
1923–

From *Catch-22*
[*The Texan*]

IT was love at first sight.

The first time Yossarian saw the chaplain he fell madly in love with him.

Yossarian was in the hospital with a pain in his liver that fell just short of being jaundice. The doctors were puzzled by the fact that it wasn't quite jaundice. If it became jaundice they could treat it. If it didn't become jaundice and went away they could discharge him. But this just being short of jaundice all the time confused them.

Each morning they came around, three brisk and serious men with efficient mouths and inefficient eyes, accompanied by brisk and serious Nurse Duckett, one of the ward nurses who didn't like Yossarian. They read the chart at the foot of the bed and asked impatiently about the pain. They seemed irritated when he told them it was exactly the same.

'Still no movement?' the full colonel demanded.

The doctors exchanged a look when he shook his head.

'Give him another pill.'

Nurse Duckett made a note to give Yossarian another pill, and the four of them moved along to the next bed. None of the nurses liked Yossarian. Actually, the pain in his liver had gone away, but Yossarian didn't say anything and the doctors never suspected. They just suspected that he had been moving his bowels and not telling anyone.

Yossarian had everything he wanted in the hospital. The food wasn't too bad, and his meals were brought to him in bed. There were extra rations of fresh meat, and during the hot part of the afternoon he and the others were served chilled fruit juice or chilled chocolate milk. Apart from the doctors and the nurses, no one ever disturbed him. For a little while in the morning he had to censor letters, but he was free after that to spend the rest of each day lying around idly with a clear conscience. He was comfortable in the hospital, and it was easy to stay on because he always ran a temperature of 101. He was even more comfortable than Dunbar, who had to keep falling down on his face in order to get *his* meals brought to him in bed.

After he had made up his mind to spend the rest of the war in the hospital, Yossarian wrote letters to everyone he knew saying that he was in the hospital but never mentioning why. One day he had a better idea. To everyone he knew he wrote that he was going on a very dangerous mission. 'They asked for volunteers. It's very dangerous, but someone has to do it. I'll write you the instant I get back.' And he had not written anyone since.

All the officer patients in the ward were forced to censor letters written by all the enlisted-men patients, who were kept in residence in wards of their own. It was a monotonous job, and Yossarian was disappointed to learn that the lives of enlisted men were only slightly more interesting than the lives of officers. After the first day he had no curiosity at all. To break the monotony he invented games. Death to all modifiers, he declared one day, and out of every letter that passed through his hands went every adverb and every adjective. The next day he made war on articles. He reached a much higher plane of creativity the following day when he blacked out everything in the letters but *a*, *an* and *the*. That erected more dynamic intralinear tensions, he felt, and in just about every case left a message far more universal. Soon he was proscribing parts of salutations and signatures and leaving the text untouched. One time he blacked out all but the salutation 'Dear Mary' from a letter, and at the bottom he wrote, 'I yearn for you tragically. R. O. Shipman, Chaplain, U.S. Army.' R. O. Shipman was the group chaplain's name.

When he had exhausted all possibilities in the letters, he began attacking the names and addresses on the envelopes, obliterating whole homes and streets, annihilating entire metropolises with careless flicks of his wrist as though he were God. Catch-22 required that each censored letter bear the censoring officer's name. Most letters he didn't read at all. On those he didn't read at all he wrote his own name. On those he did read he wrote, 'Washington Irving'. When that grew monotonous he wrote, 'Irving Washington'. Censoring the envelopes had serious repercussions, produced a ripple of anxiety on some ethereal military echelon that floated a CID man back into the ward posing as a patient. They all knew he was a CID man because he kept inquiring about an officer named Irving or Washington and because after his first day there he wouldn't censor letters. He found them too monotonous.

It was a good ward this time, one of the best he and Dunbar had ever enjoyed. With them this time was the 24-year-old fighter-pilot captain with the sparse golden mustache who had been shot into the Adriatic Sea in midwinter and not even caught cold. Now the summer was upon them, the captain had not been shot down, and he said he had the grippe. In the bed on Yossarian's right, still lying amorously on his belly, was the startled captain with malaria in his blood and a mosquito bite on his ass. Across the aisle from Yossarian was Dunbar, and next to Dunbar was the artillery captain with whom Yossarian had stopped playing chess. The captain was a good chess player, and the games were always interesting. Yossarian had stopped playing chess with him because the games were so interesting they were foolish. Then there was the educated Texan from Texas who looked like someone in Technicolor and felt, patriotically, that people of means—decent folk—should be given more votes than drifters, whores, criminals, degenerates, atheists, and indecent folk—people without means.

Yossarian was unspringing rhythms in the letters the day they brought the Texan in. It was another quiet, hot, untroubled day. The heat pressed heavily on the roof, stifling sound. Dunbar was lying motionless on his back again with his eyes staring up at the ceiling like a doll's. He was working hard at increasing his life span. He did it by cultivating boredom. Dunbar was working so hard at increasing his life span that Yossarian thought he was dead. They put the Texan in a bed in the middle of the ward, and it wasn't long before he donated his views.

Dunbar sat up like a shot. 'That's it,' he cried excitedly. 'There was something missing—all the time I knew there was something missing—and now I know what it is.' He banged his fist down into his palm. 'No patriotism,' he declared.

'You're right,' Yossarian shouted back. 'You're right, you're right, you're right.

The hot dog, the Brooklyn Dodgers. Mom's apple pie. That's what everyone's fighting for. But who's fighting for the decent folk? Who's fighting for more votes for the decent folk? There's no patriotism, that's what it is. And no matriotism, either.'

The warrant officer on Yossarian's left was unimpressed. 'Who gives a shit?' he asked tiredly, and turned over on his side to go to sleep.

The Texan turned out to be good-natured, generous, and likable. In three days no one could stand him.

He sent shudders of annoyance scampering up ticklish spines, and everybody fled from him—everybody but the soldier in white, who had no choice. The soldier in white was encased from head to toe in plaster and gauze. He had two useless legs and two useless arms. He had been smuggled into the ward during the night, and the men had no idea he was among them until they awoke in the morning and saw the two strange legs hoisted from the hips, the two strange arms anchored up perpendicularly, all four limbs pinioned strangely in air by lead weights suspended darkly above him that never moved. Sewn into the bandages over the insides of both elbows were zippered lips through which he was fed clear fluid from a clear jar. A silent zinc pipe rose from the cement on his groin and was coupled to a slim rubber hose that carried waste from his kidneys and dripped it efficiently into a clear, stoppered jar on the floor. When the jar on the floor was full, the jar feeding his elbow was empty, and the two were simply switched quickly so that the stuff could drip back into him. All they ever really saw of the soldier in white was a frayed black hole over his mouth.

The soldier in white had been filed next to the Texan, and the Texan sat sideways on his own bed and talked to him throughout the morning, afternoon, and evening in a pleasant, sympathetic drawl. The Texan never minded that he got no reply.

Temperatures were taken twice a day in the ward. Early each morning and late each afternoon Nurse Cramer entered with a jar full of thermometers and worked her way up one side of the ward and down the other, distributing a thermometer to each patient. She managed the soldier in white by inserting a thermometer into the hole over his mouth and leaving it balanced there on the lower rim. When she returned to the man in the first bed, she took his thermometer and recorded his temperature, and then moved on to the next bed and continued around the ward again. One afternoon when she had completed her first circuit of the ward and came a second time to the soldier in white, she read his thermometer and discovered that he was dead.

'Murderer,' Dunbar said quietly.

The Texan looked up at him with an uncertain grin.

'Killer,' Yossarian said.

'What are you fellas talkin' about?' the Texan asked nervously.

'You murdered him,' said Dunbar.

'You killed him,' said Yossarian.

The Texan shrank back. 'You fellas are crazy. I didn't even touch him.'

'You murdered him,' said Dunbar.

'I heard you kill him,' said Yossarian.

'You killed him because he was a nigger,' Dunbar said.

'You fellas are crazy,' the Texan cried. 'They don't allow niggers in here. They got a special place for niggers.'

'The sergeant smuggled him in,' Dunbar said.

'The Communist sergeant,' said Yossarian.

'And you knew it.'

The warrant officer on Yossarian's left was unimpressed by the entire incident of the soldier in white. The warrant officer was unimpressed by everything and never spoke at all unless it was to show irritation.

The day before Yossarian met the chaplain, a stove exploded in the mess hall and set fire to one side of the kitchen. An intense heat flashed through the area. Even in Yossarian's ward, almost three hundred feet away, they could hear the roar of the blaze and the sharp cracks of flaming timber. Smoke sped past the orange-tinted windows. In about fifteen minutes the crash trucks from the airfield arrived to fight the fire. For a frantic half hour it was touch and go. Then the firemen began to get the upper hand. Suddenly there was the monotonous old drone of bombers returning from a mission, and the firemen had to roll up their hoses and speed back to the field in case one of the planes crashed and caught fire. The planes landed safely. As soon as the last one was down, the firemen wheeled their trucks around and raced back up the hill to resume their fight with the fire at the hospital. When they got there, the blaze was out. It had died of its own accord, expired completely without even an ember to be watered down, and there was nothing for the disappointed firemen to do but drink tepid coffee and hang around trying to screw the nurses.

The chaplain arrived the day after the fire. Yossarian was busy expurgating all but romance words from the letters when the chaplain sat down in a chair between the beds and asked him how he was feeling. He had placed himself a bit to one side, and the captain's bars on the tab of his shirt collar were all the insignia Yossarian could see. Yossarian had no idea who he was and just took it for granted that he was either another doctor or another madman.

'Oh, pretty good,' he answered. 'I've got a slight pain in my liver and I haven't been the most regular of fellows, I guess, but all in all I must admit that I feel pretty good.'

'That's good,' said the chaplain.

'Yes,' Yossarian said. 'Yes, that is good.'

'I meant to come around sooner,' the chaplain said, 'but I really haven't been well.'

'That's too bad,' Yossarian said.

'Just a head cold,' the chaplain added quickly.

'I've got a fever of a hundred and one,' Yossarian added just as quickly.

'That's too bad,' said the chaplain.

'Yes,' Yossarian agreed. 'Yes, that is too bad.'

The chaplain fidgeted. 'Is there anything I can do for you?' he asked after a while.

'No, no.' Yossarian sighed. 'The doctors are doing all that's humanly possible, I suppose.'

'No, no.' The chaplain colored faintly. 'I didn't mean anything like that. I meant cigarettes . . . or books . . . or . . . toys.'

'No, no,' Yossarian said. 'Thank you. I have everything I need, I suppose—everything but good health.'

'That's too bad.'

'Yes,' Yossarian said. 'Yes, that is too bad.'

The chaplain stirred again. He looked from side to side a few times, then gazed up at the ceiling, then down at the floor. He drew a deep breath.

'Lieutenant Nately sends his regards,' he said.

Yossarian was sorry to hear they had a mutual friend. It seemed there was a basis to their conversation after all. 'You know Lieutenant Nately?' he asked regretfully.

'Yes, I know Lieutenant Nately quite well.'

'He's a bit loony, isn't he?'

The chaplain's smile was embarrassed. 'I'm afraid I couldn't say. I don't think I know him that well'.

'You can take my word for it,' Yossarian said. 'He's as goofy as they come.'

The chaplain weighed the next silence heavily and then shattered it with an abrupt question. 'You are Captain Yossarian, aren't you?'

'Nately had a bad start. He came from a good family.'

'Please excuse me,' the chaplain persisted timorously. 'I may be committing a very grave error. Are you Captain Yossarian?'

'Yes,' Captain Yossarian confessed. 'I am Captain Yossarian.'

'Of the 256th Squadron?'

'Of the fighting 256th Squadron,' Yossarian replied. 'I didn't know there were any other Captain Yossarians. As far as I know, I'm the only Captain Yossarian I know, but that's only as far as I know.'

'I see,' the chaplain said unhappily.

'That's two to the fighting eighth power,' Yossarian pointed out, 'if you're thinking of writing a symbolic poem about our squadron.'

'No,' mumbled the chaplain. 'I'm not thinking of writing a symbolic poem about your squadron.'

Yossarian straightened sharply when he spied the tiny silver cross on the other side of the chaplain's collar. He was thoroughly astonished, for he had never really talked with a chaplain before.

'You're a chaplain,' he exclaimed ecstatically. 'I didn't know you were a chaplain.'

'Why, yes,' the chaplain answered. 'Didn't you know I was a chaplain?'

'Why, no. I didn't know you were a chaplain.' Yossarian stared at him with a big, fascinated grin. 'I've never really seen a chaplain before.'

The chaplain flushed again and gazed down at his hands. He was a slight man of about 32 with tan hair and brown diffident eyes. His face was narrow and rather pale. An innocent nest of ancient pimple pricks lay in the basin of each cheek. Yossarian wanted to help him.

'Can I do anything at all to help you?' the chaplain asked.

'Yossarian shook his head, still grinning. 'No, I'm sorry. I have everything I need and I'm quite comfortable. In fact, I'm not even sick.'

'That's good.' As soon as the chaplain said the words, he was sorry and shoved his knuckles into his mouth with a giggle of alarm, but Yossarian remained silent and disappointed him. 'There are other men in the group I must visit,' he apologized finally. 'I'll come to see you again, probably tomorrow.'

'Please do that,' Yossarian said.

'I'll come only if you want me to,' the chaplain said, lowering his head shyly. 'I've noticed that I make many of the men uncomfortable.'

Yossarian glowed with affection. 'I want you to,' he said. 'You won't make me uncomfortable.'

The chaplain beamed gratefully and then peered down at a slip of paper he had been concealing in his hand all the while. He counted along the beds in the ward, moving his lips, and then centered his attention dubiously on Dunbar.

'May I inquire,' he whispered softly, 'if that is Lieutenant Dunbar?'

'Yes,' Yossarian answered loudly, 'that is Lieutenant Dunbar.'

'Thank you,' the chaplain whispered. 'Thank you very much. I must visit with him. I must visit with every member of the group who is in the hospital.'

'Even those in the other wards?' Yossarian asked.

'Even those in the other wards.'

'Be careful in those other wards, Father,' Yossarian warned. 'That's where they keep the mental cases. They're filled with lunatics.'

'It isn't necessary to call me Father,' the chaplain explained. 'I'm an Anabaptist.'

'I'm dead serious about those other wards,' Yossarian continued grimly. 'MPs won't protect you, because they're craziest of all. I'd go with you myself, but I'm scared stiff. Insanity is contagious. This is the only sane ward in the whole hospital. Everybody is crazy but us. This is probably the only sane ward in the whole world, for that matter.'

The chaplain rose quickly and edged away from Yossarian's bed, and then nodded with a conciliating smile and promised to conduct himself with appropriate caution. 'And now I must visit with Lieutenant Dunbar,' he said. Still he lingered, remorsefully. 'How is Lieutenant Dunbar?' he asked at last.

'As good as they go,' Yossarian assured him. 'A true prince. One of the finest, least dedicated men in the whole world.'

'I didn't mean that,' the chaplain answered, whispering again. 'Is he very sick?'

'No, he isn't very sick. In fact, he isn't sick at all.'

'That's good.' The chaplain sighed with relief.

'Yes,' Yossarian said. 'Yes, that is good.'

'A chaplain,' Dunbar said when the chaplain had visited him and gone. 'Did you see that? A chaplain.'

'Wasn't he sweet?' said Yossarian. 'Maybe they should give him three votes.'

'Who's they?' Dunbar demanded suspiciously.

In a bed in the small private section at the end of the ward, always working ceaselessly behind the green plyboard partition, was the solemn middle-aged colonel who was visited everyday by a gentle, sweet-faced woman with curly ash-blond hair who was not a nurse and not a Wac and not a Red Cross girl but who nevertheless appeared faithfully at the hospital in Pianosa each afternoon wearing pretty pastel summer dresses that were very smart and white leather pumps with heels half high at the base of nylon seams that were inevitably straight. The colonel was in Communications, and he was kept busy day and night transmitting glutinous messages from the interior into square pads of gauze which he sealed meticulously and delivered to a covered white pail that stood on the night table beside his bed. The colonel was gorgeous. He had a cavernous mouth, cavernous cheeks, cavernous, sad, mildewed eyes. His face was the color of clouded silver. He coughed quietly, gingerly, and dabbed the pads slowly at his lips with a distaste that had become automatic.

The colonel dwelt in a vortex of specialists who were still specializing in trying to determine what was troubling him. They hurled lights in his eyes to see if he could see, rammed needles into nerves to hear if he could feel. There was a urologist for his urine, a lymphologist for his lymph, an endocrinologist for his endocrines, a psychologist for his psyche, a dermatologist for his derma; there was a pathologist for his pathos, a cystologist for his cysts, and a bald and pedantic cetologist from the zoology department at Harvard who had been shanghaied ruthlessly into the Medical Corps by a faulty anode in an IBM machine and spent his sessions with the dying colonel trying to discuss *Moby Dick* with him.

The colonel had really been investigated. There was not an organ of his body that had not been drugged and derogated, dusted and dredged, fingered and photographed, removed, plundered and replaced. Neat, slender, and erect, the woman touched him often as she sat by his bedside and was the epitome of stately sorrow each time she smiled. The colonel was tall, thin, and stooped. When he rose to walk, he bent forward even more, making a deep cavity of his body, and placed his feet down very carefully, moving ahead by inches from the knees down. There were violet pools under his eyes. The woman spoke softly, softer than the colonel coughed, and none of the men in the ward ever heard her voice.

In less than ten days the Texan cleared the ward. The artillery captain broke first, and after that the exodus started. Dunbar, Yossarian, and the fighter captain all bolted the same morning. Dunbar stopped having dizzy spells, and the fighter captain blew his nose. Yossarian told the doctors that the pain in his liver had gone away. It was as easy as that. Even the warrant officer fled. In less than ten days, the Texan drove everybody in the ward back to duty—everybody but the CID man, who had caught cold from the fighter captain and come down with pneumonia.

Management

Anonymous
20th Century

Socrates Inquires

SOCRATES. Do you think it right Aristodemus, that the State should concern itself with the health of the people?

ARISTODEMUS. Certainly, Socrates.

SOCRATES. And will it do this better if one man is responsible for dealing with health, or many?

ARISTODEMUS. One man, Socrates.

SOCRATES. I suppose that this man, then, should be someone who himself knows about health and sickness?

ARISTODEMUS. By no means, Socrates. In my view he will look after the health of the people better if he knows nothing about it.

SOCRATES. Why do you think that, Aristodemus?

ARISTODEMUS. The man who knows something about health and sickness will have ideas about these subjects, and so he will not come to his task with an open mind.

SOCRATES. He should not be a doctor then?

ARISTODEMUS. Certainly not.

SOCRATES. You would not see the same objection to a lawyer?

ARISTODEMUS. No, on the contrary, a lawyer would be very suitable.

SOCRATES. But after a time, I suppose, the lawyer would begin to know something about health and sickness. Would he not then become disqualified for his task?

ARISTODEMUS. When that happens, Socrates, he should be moved to another post, and another man who is completely ignorant of the subject appointed to succeed him.

SOCRATES. But if the man responsible for health knows nothing about the subject, I suppose he must have advisers who do.

ARISTODEMUS. Certainly, Socrates, but again we must be careful that they are as ignorant of health as is practicable.

SOCRATES. Will they not be doctors then?

ARISTODEMUS. There must be some doctors, but we must see that they are subordinated to the laymen.

SOCRATES. But these laymen, no doubt, will have special knowledge of health and sickness so far as a layman can?

ARISTODEMUS. On the contrary, Socrates, it is important that they should have been trained in other work, especially the Treasury.

SOCRATES. But the doctors who advise the laymen will at least themselves have special knowledge of health and sickness?

ARISTODEMUS. They must be carefully chosen, Socrates, so that they have as little knowledge as possible of the work they are to do. If the State has to concern itself much with those doctors who spend their time treating the sick, the most suitable doctors to organize this will be those who have experience of preventing epidemics.

SOCRATES. Tell me, Glauco, do you share the views of Aristodemus?

GLAUCO. Every sensible man must share them, Socrates, but he has not stated all the reasons why those responsible for the health of the people should as far as possible be ignorant of the subject. In a democracy the consumer is a most important person, and the man responsible for the health of the people should represent the consumer of medicine, that is the patient; and he will necessarily be ignorant of medicine.

SOCRATES. Is the consumer the person for whose benefit a commodity is produced, or a service rendered?

GLAUCO. That is so, Socrates.

SOCRATES. Who then is the consumer of the Law? Is not the criminal such a consumer? And would you say that a criminal should be responsible for administering the Law?

GLAUCO. You are joking, Socrates! For a criminal to administer the Law would contradict its purpose!

SOCRATES. Well, then, at least the Law exists to serve every citizen?

GLAUCO. Certainly.

SOCRATES. So if you are right, an ordinary citizen should administer the Law rather than a lawyer.

GLAUCO. I suppose so, Socrates.

SOCRATES. And a doctor's knowledge of Medicine would not disqualify him from this?

GLAUCO. No indeed.

SOCRATES. So if it is fitting that a lawyer should be responsible to the State for the health of the people, would it not also be fitting that a doctor should be the chief administrator of the Law?

GLAUCO. It would seem so, Socrates.

APOLLODORUS. But Socrates, as a lawyer, I cannot agree with that! The Law occupies a unique position in the State. It is the regulator of all those relations between individuals upon which Society depends. That is why a lawyer is the best man to be the head of any inquiry which concerns the welfare of the State or its citizens.

SOCRATES. If the Law is thus all-embracing is it not important that its administration should be kept separate from politics?

APOLLODORUS. Yes.

SOCRATES. And that those who make the laws and those who administer them should be different persons?

APPOLODORUS. I agree.

SOCRATES. It would follow, would it not, that the head of the Law should not be a lawmaker nor a politician.

APOLLODORUS. In principle, perhaps, but in practice the uniqueness of the lawyer makes it easy for him to combine all these activities to their mutual advantage.

SOCRATES. Well then if, apart from Law, expert knowledge disqualifies a man from administration, so that a doctor ought not to be responsible for the health of the people, for what task in the State is a doctor fitted?

ARISTODEMUS. Since a doctor is not allowed to advertise himself he is specially qualified for a task involving advertisement. A doctor should be appointed, Socrates, to proclaim the virtues of Government. He should be a Stentor for the State.

⇥5⇤
Healing

*T*HE *idea of healing has never been completely medicalized. It is true that the surgeon's knife can be called healing, but even surgeons will allow that whereas cutting may sometimes be necessary for healing it is never sufficient. This is because we are aware that healing involves our minds and our feelings—our spirits—as well as our bodies. Indeed, it is perfectly natural to go along with Handel and allow that music can heal our sadness. This section records a few of the many ways—operations, taking the waters, spells, painting, music—in which human beings have pursued healing.*

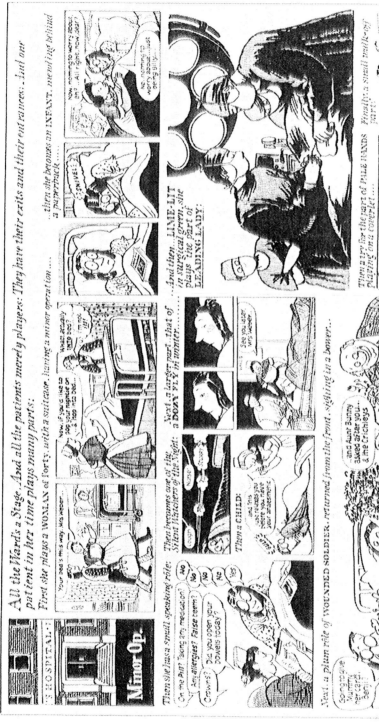

Operations

Fanny Burney
(Mme d'Arblay)
1752–1840

From *a Letter to her Sister on a Mastectomy*

M. DUBOIS now tried to issue his commands *en militaire*, but I resisted all that were resistable—I was compelled, however, to submit to taking off my long robe de Chambre, which I had meant to retain—Ah, then, how did I think of My Sisters!—not one, at so dreadful an instant, at hand, to protect—adjust—guard me . . .—My distress was, I suppose, apparent, though not my Wishes, for M. Dubois himself now softened, & spoke soothingly. Can *You*, I cried, feel for an operation that, to *You*, must seem so trivial?—Trivial? he repeated—taking up a bit of paper, which he tore, unconsciously, into a million of pieces, 'oui—*c'est peu de chose*— *mais—*' he stammered, & could not go on. No one else attempted to speak, but I was softened myself, when I saw even M. Dubois grow agitated, while Dr Larry kept always aloof, yet a glance shewed me he was pale as ashes. I knew not, positively, then, the immediate danger, but everything convinced me danger was hovering about me, & that this experiment could alone save me from its jaws. I mounted, therefore, unbidden, the Bed stead—& M. Dubois placed me upon the Mattress, & spread a cambric handkerchief upon my face. It was transparent, however, & I saw, through it, that the Bed stead was instantly surrounded by the 7 men & my nurse. I refused to be held; but when, Bright through the cambric, I saw the glitter of polished Steel—I closed my Eyes. I would not trust to convulsive fear the sight of the terrible incision. A silence the most profound ensued, which lasted for some minutes, during which, I imagine, they took their orders by signs, & made their examination—Oh what a horrible suspension!—I did not breathe—&

M. Dubois tried vainly to find any pulse. This pause, at length, was broken by Dr. Larry, who, in a voice of solemn melancholy, said 'Qui me tiendra ce sein?—'

No one answered; at least not verbally; but this aroused me from my passively submissive state, for I feared they imagined the whole breast infected—feared it too justly,—for, again through the Cambric, I saw the hand of M. Dubois held up, while his fore finger first described a straight line from top to bottom of the breast, secondly a Cross, & thirdly a circle; intimating that the WHOLE was to be taken off. Excited by this idea, I started up, threw off my veil, &, in answer to the demand 'Qui me tiendra ce sein?', cried 'C'est moi, Monsieur!' & I held My hand under it, & explained the nature of my sufferings, which all sprang from one point, though they darted into every part. I was heard attentively, but in utter silence, & M. Dubois then re-placed me as before, &, as before, spread my veil over my face. How vain, alas, my representation! immediately again I saw the fatal finger describe the Cross—& the circle—Hopeless, then, desperate, & self-given up, I closed once more my Eyes, relinquishing all watching, all resistance, all interference, & sadly resolute to be wholly resigned.

My dearest Esther,—& all my dears to whom she communicates this doleful ditty, will rejoice to hear that this resolution once taken, was firmly adhered to, in defiance of a terror that surpasses all description, & the most torturing pain. Yet— when the dreadful steel was plunged into the breast—cutting through veins— arteries—flesh—nerves—I needed no injunctions not to restrain my cries. I began a scream that lasted unintermittingly during the whole time of the incision—& I almost marvel that it rings not in my Ears still! so excruciating was the agony. When the wound was made, & the instrument was withdrawn, the pain seemed undiminished, for the air that suddenly rushed into those delicate parts felt like a mass of minute but sharp & forked poniards, that were tearing the edges of the wound—but when again I felt the instrument—describing a curve—cutting against the grain, if I may so say, while the flesh resisted in a manner so forcible as to oppose & tire the hand of the operator, who was forced to change from the right to the left—then, indeed, I thought I must have expired. I attempted no more to open my Eyes,—they felt as if hermetically shut, & so firmly closed, that the Eyelids seemed indented into the Cheeks. The instrument this second time withdrawn, I concluded the operation over—Oh no! presently the terrible cutting was renewed—& worse than ever, to separate the bottom, the foundation of this dreadful gland from the parts to which it adhered—Again all description would be baffled—yet again all was not over,—Dr Larry rested but his own hand, &—Oh Heaven!—I then felt the Knife ⟨rack⟩ling against the breast bone—scraping it!—

This performed, while I yet remained in utterly speechless torture, I heard the Voice of Mr Larry,—(all others guarded a dead silence) in a tone nearly tragic, desire everyone present to pronounce if anything more remained to be done. The general voice was Yes,—but the finger of Mr Dubois—which I literally *felt* elevated over the wound, though I saw nothing, & though he touched nothing, so indescribably sensitive was the spot—pointed to some further requisition—& again began the scraping!—and, after this, Dr Moreau thought he discerned a peccant atom—and still, & still, M. Dubois demanded atom after atom . . .

To conclude, the evil was so profound, the case so delicate, & the precautions necessary for preventing a return so numerous, that the operation, including the treatment & the dressing, lasted 20 minutes! a time, for sufferings so acute, that was hardly supportable—However, I bore it with all the courage I could exert, & never moved, nor stopt them, nor resisted, nor remonstrated, nor spoke—except once or twice, during the dressings, to say 'Ah Messieurs! que je vous plains!—' for indeed I was sensible to the feeling concern with which they all saw what I endured, though my speech was principally—*very* principally meant for Dr Larry. Except this, I uttered not a syllable, save, when so often they recommenced, calling out 'Avertissez moi, Messieurs! avertissez moi!—' Twice, I believe, I fainted; at least, I have two total chasms in my memory of this transaction, that impede my tying together what passed. When all was done, & they lifted me up that I might be put to bed, my strength was so totally annihilated, that I was obliged to be carried, & could not even sustain my hands & arms, which hung as if I had been lifeless; while my face, as the Nurse has told me, was utterly colourless. This removal made me open my Eyes—& I then saw my good Dr Larry, pale nearly as myself, his face streaked with blood, & its expression depicting grief, apprehension, & almost horrour. *She ended the letter: 'I am at this moment quite Well . . . Read, therefore, this Narrative at your leisure, & without emotion—for all has ended happily.'*

[*Editor's Note:* Fanny Burney lived for many years after this operation.]

James Kirkup
1918–

A Correct Compassion

(To Mr Philip Allison, after watching him perform a Mitral Stenosis Valvulotomy in the General Infirmary at Leeds.)

CLEANLY, sir, you went to the core of the matter.
Using the purest kind of wit, a balance of belief and art,
You with a curious nervous elegance laid bare
The root of life, and put your finger on its beating heart.

The glistening theatre swarms with eyes, and hands, and eyes,
On green-clothed tables, ranks of instruments transmit a sterile gleam.
The masks are on, and no unnecessary smile betrays
A certain tension, true concomitant of calm.

Here we communicate by looks, though words,
Too, are used, as in continuous historic present
You describe our observations and your deeds.
All gesture is reduced to its result, an instrument.

She who does not know she is a patient lies
Within a tent of green, and sleeps without a sound
Beneath the lamps, and the reflectors that devise
Illuminations probing the profoundest wound.

A calligraphic master, improvising, you invent
The first incision, and no poet's hesitation
Before his snow-blank page mars your intent:
The flowing stroke is drawn like an uncalculated inspiration.

A garland of flowers unfurls across the painted flesh.
With quick precision the arterial forceps click.
Yellow threads are knotted with a simple flourish.
Transfused, the blood preserves its rose, though it is sick.

Meters record the blood, measure heart-beats, control the breath.
Hieratic gesture: scalpel bares a creamy rib; with pincer knives
The bone quietly is clipped, and lifted out. Beneath,
The pink, black-mottled lung like a revolted creature heaves,

Collapses; as if by extra fingers is neatly held aside
By two ordinary egg-beaters, kitchen tools that curve
Like extraordinary hands. Heart, laid bare, silently beats. It can hide
No longer, yet is not revealed.—'A local anaesthetic in the cardiac nerve.'

Now, in firm hands that quiver with a careful strength,
Your knife feels through the heart's transparent skin; at first,
Inside the pericardium, slit down half its length,
The heart, black-veined, swells like a fruit about to burst,

But goes on beating, love's poignant image bleeding at the dart
Of a more grievous passion, as a bird, dreaming of flight, sleeps on
Within its leafy cage.—'It generally upsets the heart
A bit, though not unduly, when I make the first injection.'

Still, still the patient sleeps, and still the speaking heart is dumb.
The watchers breathe an air far sweeter, rarer than the room's.
The cold walls listen. Each in his own blood hears the drum
She hears, tented in green, unfathomable calms.

'I make a purse-string suture here, with a reserve
Suture, which I must make first, and deeper,
As a safeguard, should the other burst. In the cardiac nerve
I inject again a local anaesthetic. Could we have fresh towels to cover

All these adventitious ones. Now can you all see?
When I put my finger inside the valve, there may be a lot
Of blood, and it may come with quite a bang. But I let it flow,
In case there are any clots, to give the heart a good clean-out.

Now can you give me every bit of light you've got.'
We stand on the benches, peering over his shoulder.
The lamp's intensest rays are concentrated on an inmost heart.
Someone coughs.—'If you have to cough, you will do it outside this
theatre.'— 'Yes, sir.'

'How's she breathing, Doug? Do you feel quite happy?'—'Yes, fairly
Happy.'—'Now. I am putting my finger in the opening of the valve.
I can only get the tip of my finger in.—It's gradually
Giving way.—I'm inside.—No clots.—I can feel the valve

Breathing freely now around my finger, and the heart working.
Not too much blood. It opened very nicely.
I should say that anatomically speaking
This is a perfect case.—Anatomically.

For, of course, anatomy is not physiology.'
We find we breathe again, and hear the surgeon hum.
Outside, in the street, a car starts up. The heart regularly
Thunders.—'I do not stitch up the pericardium.

It is not necessary.'—For this is imagination's other place,
Where only necessary things are done, with the supreme and grave
Dexterity that ignores technique; with proper grace
Informing a correct compassion, that performs its love, and makes it
live.

Miroslav Holub
1923–

Heart Transplant

AFTER an hour

there's an abyss in the chest
created by the missing heart
like a model landscape
where humans have grown extinct.

The drums of extracorporeal circulation
introduce
an inaudible
New World Symphony.

It's like falling from an aeroplane, the air growing
    cooler and cooler,
until it condenses in the inevitable moonlight,
the clouds coming closer, below the left foot, below
    the right foot,
a microscopic landscape with roads like capillaries
pulsing in counter-movements,
feeble hands grasping for the King of Blood,
'Seek the Lord while he may be found,'
ears ringing with the whistles of some kind of cosmic
    marmots,
an indifferent bat's membrane spreading between the
    nerves,
'It is unworthy of great hearts to broadcast their own
    confusion.'

It's like falling from an aeroplane
before the masked face of a creator
who's dressed in a scrub suit
and latex gloves.

Now they are bringing, bedded in melting ice,
the new heart,
like some trophy
from the Eightieth Olympiad of Calamities.

Atrium is sewn to atrium,
aorta to aorta,
three hours of eternity
coming and going.

And when the heart begins to beat
and the curves jump
like synthetic sheep
on a green screen,
it's like a model of a battlefield
where Life and Spirit have been fighting

and both have won.

(Translated from the Czech by David Young and Dana Hábová)

Dannie Abse
1926–

In the Theatre

(A true incident)

'Only a local anaesthetic was given because of the blood pressure problem. The patient, thus, was fully awake throughout the operation. But in those days—in 1938, in Cardiff, when I was Lambert Rogers' dresser—they could not locate a brain tumour with precision. Too much normal brain tissue was destroyed as the surgeon crudely searched for it, before he felt the resistance of it . . . all somewhat hit and miss. One operation I shall never forget. . . .'
                                              (Dr Wilfred Abse)

SISTER saying—'Soon you'll be back in the ward,'
sister thinking—'Only two more on the list,'
the patient saying—'Thank you, I feel fine';
small voices, small lies, nothing untoward,
though, soon, he would blink again and again
because of the fingers of Lambert Rogers,
rash as a blind man's, inside his soft brain.

If items of horror can make a man laugh
then laugh at this: one hour later, the growth
still undiscovered, ticking its own wild time;
more brain mashed because of the probe's braille path;
Lambert Rogers desperate, fingering still;
his dresser thinking, 'Christ! Two more on the list,
a cisternal puncture and a neural cyst.'

Then, suddenly, the cracked record in the brain,
a ventriloquist voice that cried, 'You sod,
leave my soul alone, leave my soul alone,'—
the patient's dummy lips moving to that refrain,
the patient's eyes too wide. And, shocked,
Lambert Rogers drawing out the probe
with nurses, students, sister, petrified.

'Leave my soul alone, leave my soul alone,'
that voice so arctic and that cry so odd
had nowhere else to go—till the antique
gramophone wound down and the words began
to blur and slow, '. . . leave . . . my . . . soul . . . alone . . .'
to cease at last when something other died.
And silence matched the silence under snow.

Cures

R. S. Thomas
1913–

The Cure

BUT what to do? Doctors in verse
Being scarce now, most poets
Are their own patients, compelled to treat
Themselves first, their complaint being
Peculiar always. Consider, you,
Whose rough hands manipulate
The fine bones of a sick culture,
What areas of that infirm body
Depend solely on a poet's cure.

Tobias Smollett
1721–1771

From *The Expedition of Humphry Clinker*

[*To Dr Lewis*]

Dear Dick,

I HAVE done with the waters; therefore your advice comes a day too late—I grant that physic is no mystery of your making. I know it is a mystery in its own nature; and, like other mysteries, requires a strong gulp of faith to make it go down—Two days ago, I went into the King's Bath, by the advice of our friend Ch——, in order to clear the strainer of the skin, for the benefit of a free perspiration; and the first object that saluted my eye, was a child full of scrophulous ulcers, carried in the arms of one of the guides, under the very noses of the bathers. I was so shocked at the sight, that I retired immediately with indignation and disgust—Suppose the matter of those ulcers, floating on the water, comes in contact with my skin, when the pores are all open, I would ask you what must be the consequence?—Good Heaven, the very thought makes my blood run cold! we know not what sores may be running into the water while we are bathing, and what sort of matter we may thus imbibe; the king's-evil, the scurvy, the cancer, and the pox; and, no doubt, the heat will render the *virus* the more volatile and penetrating. To purify myself from all such contamination, I went to the duke of Kingston's private Bath, and there I was almost suffocated for want of free air; the place was so small, and the steam so stifling.

After all, if the intention is no more than to wash the skin, I am convinced that simple element is more effectual than any water impregnated with salt and iron; which, being astringent, will certainly contract the pores, and leave a kind of crust upon the surface of the body. But I am now as much afraid of drinking, as of bathing; for, after a long conversation with the Doctor, about the construction of the pump and the cistern, it is very far from being clear with me, that the patients in the Pump-room don't swallow the scourings of the bathers. I can't help suspecting, that there is, or may be, some regurgitation from the bath into the cistern of the pump. In that case, what a delicate beverage is everyday quaffed by the drinkers; medicated with the sweat and dirt, and dandruff; and the abominable discharges of various kinds, from twenty different diseased bodies, parboiling in the kettle below. In order to avoid this filthy composition, I had recourse to the spring that supplies the private baths on the Abbey-green; but I at once perceived something extraordinary in the taste and smell; and, upon inquiry, I find that the Roman baths in this quarter, were found covered by an old burying ground, belonging to the Abbey; through which, in all probability, the water drains in its passage; so that as we drink the decoction of living bodies at the Pump-room, we swallow the strainings of rotten bones and carcasses at the private bath—I vow to God, the very idea turns my stomach!—Determined, as I am, against any farther use of the Bath waters, this consideration would give me little disturbance, if I could find anything more pure, or less pernicious, to quench my thirst; but, although the natural springs of excellent water are seen gushing spontaneous on every side, from the hills that surround us, the inhabitants, in general, make use of well-water, so impregnated with nitre, or alum, or some other villainous mineral, that it is equally ungrateful to the taste, and mischievous to the constitution. It must be owned, indeed, that here, in Milsham-street, we have a precarious and scanty supply from the hill; which is collected in an open basin in the Circus, liable to be defiled with dead dogs, cats, rats, and every species of nastiness, which the rascally populace may throw into it, from mere wantonness and brutality . . .

Yours,

Bath   Matt. Bramble

(1771)

F. W. Nietzsche
1844–1900

Health

FOR there is no health as such, and all attempts to define anything in that way have been miserable failures. Even the determination of what health means for your *body* depends on your goal, your horizon, your energies, your drives, your errors, and above all on the ideals and phantasms of your soul. Thus there are innumerable healths of the body; and . . . the more we put aside the dogma of the 'equality of men', the more must the concept of a normal health, along with a normal diet and the normal course of an illness be abandoned by our physicians. Only then would the time have come to reflect on the health and sicknesses of the *soul*, and to find the peculiar virtue of each man in the health of his soul: in one person's case this health could, of course, look like the opposite of health in another person.

(Translated from the German by W. Kaufmann)

Spells, Hope, and Mothers

Thomas Flatman
1637–1688

*On Mistress S.W., who cured my hand by a plaster
applied to the knife which hurt me*

WOUNDED and weary of my life,
I to my fair one sent my knife;
The point had pierced my hand as far
As foe would foe in open war.
Cruel, but yet compassionate, she
Spread plasters for my enemy;
She hugg'd the wretch had done me harm,
And in her bosom kept it warm,
When suddenly I found the cure was done,
The pain and all the anguish gone,
Those nerves which stiff and tender were
Now very free and active are:
Not help'd by any power above,
But a true miracle of Love.
Henceforth, physicians, burn your bills,
Prescribe no more uncertain pills:
She can at distance vanquish pain,
She makes the grave to gape in vain:
'Mongst all the arts that saving be
None so sublime as sympathy.

Oh could it help a wounded breast,
I'd send my soul to have it dress'd.
Yet, rather, let herself apply
The sovereign med'cine to her eye:
There lurks the weapon wounds me deep,
There, that which stabs me in my sleep;
For still I feel, within, a mortall smart,
The salve that heal'd my hand can't cure my heart.

Mother Goose

Four-Leaf Clover

ONE leaf for fame, one leaf for wealth,
One for a faithful lover,
And one leaf to bring glorious health,
Are all in a four-leaf clover.

Anonymous
17th Century

Charm of the Sprain

BRIDE went out
In the morning early,
With a pair of horses;
One broke his leg,
With much ado,
That was apart,
She put bone to bone,
She put flesh to flesh,
She put sinew to sinew,
She put vein to vein;
As she healed that
May I heal this.

Anonymous
17th Century

The Fairy Wort

PLUCK will I the fairy wort,
With expectation from the fairy bower,
To overcome every oppression,
As long as it be fairy wort.

Fairy wort, fairy wort,
I envy the one who has thee,
There is nothing the sun encircles,
But is to her a sure victory.

Pluck will I mine honoured plant
Plucked by the great Mary, helpful Mother of the
  people,
To cast off me every tale of scandal and flippancy,
Ill-life, ill-love, ill-luck,
Hatred, falsity, fraud and vexation,
Till I go in the cold grave beneath the sod.

Kathleen Raine
1908–

Spell of Sleep

LET him be safe in sleep
As leaves folded together
As young birds under wings
As the unopened flower.

Let him be hidden in sleep
As islands under rain,
As mountains with their clouds,
As hills in the mantle of dusk.

Let him be free in sleep
As the flowing tides of the sea,
As the travelling wind on the moor,
As the journeying stars in space.

Let him be upheld in sleep
As a cloud at rest on the air,
As sea-wrack under the waves
When the flowing tide covers all
And the shells' delicate lives
Open on the sea-floor.

Let him be healed in sleep
In quiet waters of night
In the mirroring pool of dreams
Where memory returns in peace,
Where the troubled spirit grows wise
And the heart is comforted.

David Rorie
1867–1946

The Healin' Herb

FOR ilka ill there is a cure,
Be it in root or leaf or floo'r,
An' aft-times roon aboot the door.

Tho' it grows free for a' mankind
Lang may ye seek afore ye find.

But for stark deid
There is nae remeid—
Nane.

Michael O'Donnell
1928–

Killjoy was here

WHATEVER craze may sweep the beaches this summer you can be sure a certain type of doctor will be at hand, eyes bright and pen primed, eager to publish the first condemnatory account of it. Medical censoriousness is an ancient tradition—some doctors are still uncertain whether they approve of sex—but in the 1950s it resurged powerfully with the coming of the hula hoop.

Doctors discovered that if they issued gloomy warnings about what hooping could do to the spine, not only did they get their letters in their professional journals but their names in the sort of newspapers read by their patients.

They needed little further encouragement and recently, for instance, we've had grave pronouncements about Jogger's Nipple, Break-dancing Neck, Crab-eater's Lung, Swim-goggle Headache, and Amusement Slide anaphylaxis.

And, in the index of the *New England Journal of Medicine*, which specializes in this sort of thing, you can find Cyclist's Pudendum, Dog Walker's Elbow, Space Invader's Wrist, Unicyclist's Sciatica, Jeans Folliculitis, Jogger's Kidney, Flautist's Neuropathy, and Urban Cowboy's Rhabdomyolosis—a painful nastiness in the muscles caused by riding mechanical bucking broncos in amusement arcades.

Censorious doctors seem particularly to enjoy knocking activities promoted by their heartier colleagues. There's an eagerness, for instance, in the way they record the afflictions of joggers, bombarding medical journals with reports of muscle and joint injuries, heart attacks, asthma, and amenorrhoea. Recently three punctilious Swiss physicians reported yet another jogging hazard: bird attacks by the European Buzzard (*Buteo buteo*).

With doctors revelling so brazenly in the role of gloomy killjoy, small wonder that patients are flocking to fringe medicine and beyond in search of the homely optimism that once radiated from Tannochbrae.

In the land of the cliché, prevention may be better than cure but, back in the real world, the punters warm more readily to dear old Dr Cameron than to finger-wagging Dr Snoddie. Medicine must not blind itself to the wisdom of great men like Mr Robert Robinson, who have said that they hope their doctors will keep any bad news to themselves. Optimism has always been powerful therapy and I have often seen optimistic doctors help patients fight off—even overcome—the effects of incurable disease.

Optimism also enhances a doctor's reputation. When his patients die, friends and relatives will say: 'The doctor was marvellous. He did all that was humanly possible but nature beat him in the end.' His reputation always outshines that of the medical pessimist whose patients never die 'in spite of his efforts'. Even worse, they occasionally survive in spite of his efforts.

The world is full of gleeful old fogies eager to describe how they cheated their pessimistic doctors. They wave their walking sticks and tell us proudly how, maybe 40 years before, some gloomy killjoy gave them only six months to live.

Optimism, I am convinced, is an essential component of that ephemeral quality possessed by doctors whom patients feel better for seeing, no matter what treatment is prescribed. Such doctors are often assumed to be endowed with gifts denied to their colder hearted colleagues, but 30 years of casual doctor-watching have persuaded me that the 'gift' is largely a technique. Given the right technique, today's gloomy denouncer of cream cakes, coffee, and BMX bicycles could transmogrify overnight into dear old Dr Cameron.

The best techniques are rarely written down but are passed by word of mouth within the brotherhood or handed down as heirlooms from doctor fathers to their doctor sons. The most valuable one I know was passed to me by the grandson of a distinguished Dublin physician, Richard Leeper.

Leeper's gift to his grandson went something like this: 'Never give medicine to a dying man. Always give him brandy. Everyone knows that brandy never harmed anyone but give the patient medicine and someone will say, "God forgive me if I wrong him, but the doctor's draught was the last thing the poor man took."'

Grandfather Leeper must have received that advice round about 1880 and no one knows how many generations it had passed through before it reached him. It could well have started with Hippocrates, for that quality of learning has an imperishable validity.

(From *Guardian*, 15 May 1985)

Merilee D. Karr
(dates unknown)

From *The Moment of Death*
[*Mothers*]

CAST OF CHARACTERS

NINA JONSON. first-year medical student

DR LARRY WILLIAMS. young private physician

SCENE

DR WILLIAMS' *office. Stacks of charts on the desk, a bookcase, diplomas on the wall, a grungy office coffeemaker, two chairs. End of day, the present. They enter and flop down in chairs, he at his desk, she in the side chair. He is carrying a stack of charts, plops them down on desk. The charts start to slide and they catch them and readjust the stack. He is wearing a white coat, she a white jacket. Both have stethoscopes slung around their necks. She has a lot of paraphernalia in the pockets (reflex hammers, note cards, books, penlights, etc.).*

NINA. Whew! Do you always work this hard?

DR WILLIAMS. Nahh. I call in extra patients when I have a student with me. Half the people you saw today were from Central Casting.

NINA. That would explain a lot. Every one of them came from a different movie.

DR WILLIAMS. My favourite was the musical comedy.

NINA. Mr and Mrs Primm?

DR WILLIAMS. Yeah. They're in the choir at church, their son is in a rock band, and they think if he would just join the choir he'd be easier to deal with. No wonder I can't control their blood pressure with pills.

NINA. You mean there's no pill to cure you of
  adolescent children?

DR WILLIAMS. I have a lot of pills for adolescents,
  but none for their parents. Do you want some
  coffee?

NINA. Sure. [*They find Styrofoam cups and set up
  coffee.*]

DR WILLIAMS. You know what the definition of a
  wonder drug is?

NINA. No, what?

DR WILLIAMS. You wonder how it works. [*Sorting
  through stack of charts.*] Let's see. We saw three kids
  today with the same disease, middle ear infection
  . . .

NINA. But from such different families!

DR WILLIAMS. Oh, yeah. You can take the same
  germ, give it to three different families, and come up
  with three different problems that you treat in three
  different ways. The illness equals the disease plus
  the person. [*Continuing to flip through the day's
  charts.*] Frieda Garvey needed a simple adjustment
  in her hypertension meds—let's hope she stays
  simple, since we also saw a lot of folks today farther
  down the road with hypertension . . .

NINA. Is that Mr Slaughter's original problem?

DR WILLIAMS. Yeah, he's a great example. That's
  classic heart pain, right in the middle of the chest,
  under the sternum. That's what happens when you
  don't take your blood pressure pills. It's hard to
  convince people that something they can't see or feel
  is dangerous.

NINA. If only it had a more dangerous name. Or if
  you could catch it from doing something fun, like
  having sex or eating, people might be more scared
  of it.

DR WILLIAMS. That's advanced for a medical
student. You're not supposed to think like that 'til
you're old and grey.

NINA. I'm older than I look. Can I ask you
something?

DR WILLIAMS. Sure.

NINA. We saw a little bit of everything today.
Wouldn't it be better for patients, and easier for
you, if you specialized in one thing, instead of
seeing all kinds of patients with all kinds of
problems?

DR WILLIAMS. I *do* specialize in one thing.

NINA. What's that?

DR WILLIAMS. I specialize in Everything.

NINA. Next you're going to tell me that one pill makes
you larger and one pill makes you small.

DR WILLIAMS. Doesn't it? Trust me. I'm a doctor.
My residency taught internal medicine *and*
paediatrics, *and* surgery, *and* obstetrics, and a lot of
applied psychology about how people act when
they're sick. That's everything I need.

NINA. How can you know everything? Once upon a
time you could but there's just too much to know
nowadays. I'm overwhelmed, my whole class is
overwhelmed, and it's only the first year. We think
we're going to kill someone because we can't
remember the Krebs cycle.

DR WILLIAMS. Nina, I have never killed anyone
because I couldn't remember the Krebs cycle. I
have never even inconvenienced anyone because I
couldn't remember the Krebs cycle. In two years,
when you start to take care of real people on the
wards, you can forget the Krebs cycle forever.
You're made to learn it once so you'll believe in it.

NINA. OK. I believe in it. Couldn't I have a catechism instead of an exam?

DR WILLIAMS. The reason you need to believe in it is that, 20 years from now, when some drug comes along that cures acute megalocanosis by altering the Krebs cycle, you'll use it, instead of sticking your head in the sand.

NINA. What's megalocanosis?

DR WILLIAMS. [*He pauses, with a concerned look.*] Didn't you recognize it in Mrs Beagleton today?

NINA. You mean the one that . . .? Is that one of those auto-immune conditions? Do you use steroids for it? I think we're going to have a lecture on it, next month.

DR WILLIAMS. I made it up. Don't ever be afraid to say you don't know. Or be afraid, but say it anyway.

NINA. Thanks. Sorry.

DR WILLIAMS. Forget it. So, you're right, there're a zillion things to know nowadays, an overwhelming unimaginable mass of fact. They're shovelling more of it out everyday. But, great news—you can forget most of it, because *common things are common.*

NINA. Common things are common?

DR WILLIAMS. Yeah. A statistical accident that makes the family doctor possible on this planet. On a planet where all diseases were distributed equally, you'd just have to know all the diseases. You'd need a computer to take care of a sore throat. Name the diseases we saw today.

NINA. [*Counting on her fingers.*] Ear infection, high blood pressure, lung cancer, back pain, alcoholism, normal pregnancy, ankautosis, mental illness, and diabetes.

DR WILLIAMS. Right. That's the Top Forty of medical problems. Except for the one you made up, nice try.

NINA. Foiled again.

DR WILLIAMS. Know those, because that's what you'll see over and over again, your bread and butter diseases. Then you can forget the details of the thousands of rare diseases that you'll never see, as long as you recognize when you see something that you've never seen before, and what system it's in so you can figure out who to refer it to. I can take care of 95% of what walks in the door, because common things are common.

NINA. So I don't need to learn all these diseases they're shoving at me in lecture?

DR WILLIAMS. I didn't say that. You don't know what's common and what's rare. And even if you do, the Top Forty will change by the time you're in practice. Keep trying to learn all of 'em. The ones you hear about over and over and over again will be the important ones, and they'll stick.

NINA. You make it sound so easy. Wouldn't it be more efficient and safer for every doctor just to know one part of the body thoroughly? Why should anyone try to be a generalist today?

DR WILLIAMS. One of my favourite teachers, a Dr Hughes, Hubert Hughes—you don't know him, he's dead now—used to tell me the same thing. He hated me for going into family medicine. When the family medicine department started up here, in the early 1960s, he lobbied against it. He thought that now that we know so much about diseases, and have so many weapons against them—so much more than we did when he was a student—we should teach students the intricacies of the diseases, and the wonderful, powerful, lifesaving drugs, and send them out like little soldiers to battle disease.

NINA. Yeah. What's wrong with that?

DR WILLIAMS. Nothing. For his time. For his time,

he was right. His worst nights were the nights he spent waiting up for a patient to die of some disease he felt helpless against. Which was most of them. Those three kids with little old ear infections today —kids used to die of that! Now we just give them antibiotics, and our worst problem is figuring out which antibiotic Welfare is paying for this month.

My worst nights—my worst nights now are the nights I spend waiting up for some patient to die of some disease that I understand damn well, and can't make my patients stop doing to themselves! Lung cancer, cirrhosis, heart disease, child abuse—what we call life-style diseases. In Hubert's time, people died because we were ignorant about disease. Now people die 'cuz they can't talk to their doctors.

NINA. Or their doctors can't talk to them.

DR WILLIAMS. Or their doctors can't talk to them. Right. That's why I'm a generalist. I talk to the whole patient, and I listen to the whole patient. I teach, I motivate, sometimes I manipulate a little. All right, sometimes I manipulate a lot. I help people get through things, and I treat the common diseases. People need someone like that.

NINA. How do you get to be someone like that?

DR WILLIAMS. I think we all start out that way, but it's hard to keep it up. Elaine and I had our first kid when I was in school, and I took some time off. Hubert hated me for that, too. He didn't know his kids—thought doctors, real doctors, weren't supposed to indulge in that sort of thing. Their own families. Their own lives. So Hubert was a star at difficult diagnoses, but he never understood his patients' families.

NINA. What a revolutionary idea, to treat the person first, and the disease second.

DR WILLIAMS. No. No, no, no. Uh-uh. That's no
revolution. That's what faith healers and quacks
have always done. With enviable success, I might
add. [*Wagging his finger at her.*] You keep wanting
to get away from those diseases.

NINA. A natural urge.

DR WILLIAMS. What's really revolutionary is treating
the person and the disease together at the same
time. You can't get away from those diseases.
They're not warm and fuzzy. And they're always
out there, waiting. Being friendly is not enough.
You have to know the diseases and the drugs and
the tests. But you will.

NINA. Then maybe I should get out of medicine right
now. I just failed the biochemistry exam yesterday.
I'm going to be a friendly but dumb doctor.

DR WILLIAMS. Oh. I get it, Nina. You're not dumb.
You're just overwhelmed. And you're letting the
wrong things overwhelm you. If you truly want to
get out of medicine, I can't argue. Medicine is a
dumb thing to do to your life. But don't quit for the
wrong reasons. You're not dumb. I had a dumb
student once; he scared me. You're going to be
good. You have an instinct for finding out what's
bothering your patients, and you care about them.

NINA. Me? Really?

DR WILLIAMS. Really. I would not suggest you be a
neurosurgeon . . .

NINA. Ha!

DR WILLIAMS. . . . you don't have those skills. By the
same token, I would not suggest that the
neurosurgeons be family doctors. They don't have
our skills. Look, Nina, who do you think delivers
most of the medical care in this country?

NINA. I don't know. Hospitals?

DR WILLIAMS. No. Guess again.

NINA. Health maintenance organizations.

DR WILLIAMS. Wrong.

NINA. The VA? Blue Cross?

DR WILLIAMS. Wrong again. Give up?

NINA. Yes.

DR WILLIAMS. You're sure? Don't you want another
   guess?

NINA. No! All right. I give up already!

DR WILLIAMS. Mothers. It's mothers.

[*Editor's Note*: This is an extract from a play which fulfilled Dr Karr's
'Independent Study in Medical Science' requirement when she was a fourth-year
student at the University of Washington School of Medicine, Seattle. It was
published in the *Journal of the American Medical Association*, 1968, vol. 260, no.
17.]

‭ ❧ ❧ ❦‬

Music and Art as Therapy

Robert Burton
1577–1640

Music as Therapy

MANY and sundry are the means which philosophers and physicians have prescribed to exhilarate a sorrowful heart, to divert those fixed and intent cares and meditations, which in this malady so much offend; but, in my judgement, none so present, none so powerful, none so apposite, as a cup of strong drink, mirth, music, and merry company . . . [music has the quality] not only to expel the greatest griefs, but it doth extenuate fears and furies, appeaseth cruelty, abateth heaviness; and, to such as are watchful, it causeth quiet rest; it takes away spleen and hatred, be it instrumental, vocal, with strings, wind . . . and it cures all irksomeness and heaviness of the soul. Labouring men, that sing to their work, can tell as much; and so can soldiers when they go to fight, whom terror of death cannot so much affright, as the sound of trumpet, drum, fife, and such like music animates. . . . It makes a child quiet, the nurse's song; and many times the sound of a trumpet on a sudden, bells ringing, a boy singing some ballad tune early in the street, alters, revives, recreates a restless patient that cannot sleep in the night. In a word it is so powerful a thing that it ravisheth the soul . . . the queen of the senses, by sweet pleasure (which is a happy cure:) and corporal tunes pacify our incorporeal soul . . . and carries it beyond itself, helps, elevates, extends it. Scaliger[1] gives a reason of these effects, because the spirits about the heart take in that trembling and dancing air into the body, are moved together and stirred up with it, or else the mind, as some suppose, harmonically composed, is roused up at the tunes of music. And tis not only men that are so affected, but almost all other creatures. You

---

[1] Julius Caesar Scaliger (1484–1558).

know the tale of Hercules Gailus, Orpheus, and Amphion . . . that could make stocks and stones, as well as beasts and other animals, dance after their pipes; the dog and hare, wolf and lamb . . . stood all gaping upon Orpheus; and trees, pulled up by the roots, came to hear him. . . . Anon made fishes follow him, which, as common experience evinces, are much affected with music. All singing birds are much pleased with it, especially nightingales . . . and bees among the rest, though they be flying away when they hear any tingling sound, will tarry behind. Harts, hinds, horses, dogs, bears, are exceedingly delighted with it . . .

(From *The Anatomy of Melancholy*, 1621)

Samuel Pepys
1633–1703
From *Diary*

27 February 1667. WITH my wife to the King's House to see *The Virgin Martyr*[1], the first time it hath been acted a great while; and it is mighty pleasant: not that the play is worth much, but it is finely acted by Beck Marshall. But that which did please me beyond anything in the whole world, was the wind-music when the angel came down; which is so sweet that it ravished me, and indeed, in a word, did wrap up my soul so that it made me really sick, just as I have formerly been when in love with my wife; that neither then, nor all the evening going home, and at home, I was able to think of anything but remained all night transported, so as I could not believe that ever any music hath that real command over the soul of a man as this did upon me; and makes me resolve to practice wind-music, and to make my wife do the like.

[1 A tragedy by Massinger and Dekker of 1622].

William Cowper
1731–1800

Music and Recollection

From *The Task*

THERE is in souls a sympathy with sounds,
And as the mind is pitch'd, the ear is pleased
With melting airs, or martial, brisk, or grave;
Some chord in unison with what we hear
Is touch'd within us, and the heart replies.
How soft the music of those village bells,
Falling at intervals upon the ear
In cadence sweet, now dying all away,
Now pealing loud again, and louder still,
Clear and sonorous, as the gale comes on!
With easy force it opens all the cells
Where Memory slept. Wherever I have heard
A kindred melody, the scene recurs,
And with it all its pleasures and its pains.
Such comprehensive views the spirit takes,
That in a few short moments I retrace
(As in a map the voyager his course)
The windings of my way through many years.

G. F. Handel
1685–1759

Art thou troubled?
(Dove Sei)
Aria from 'Rodelinda'

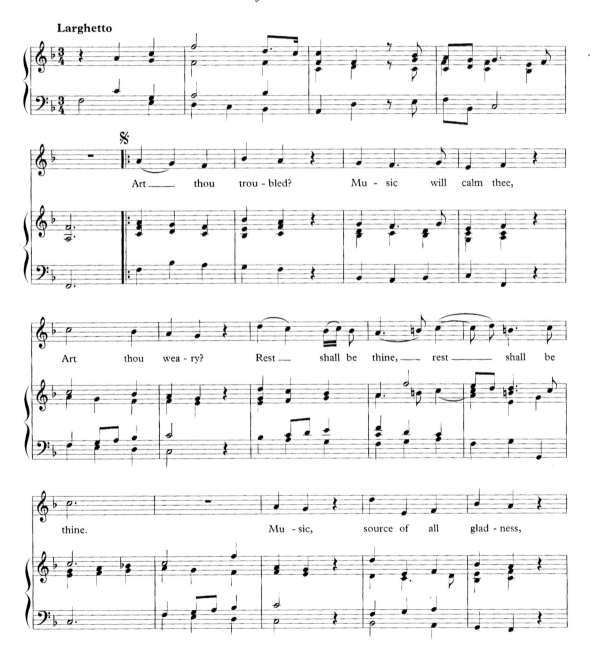

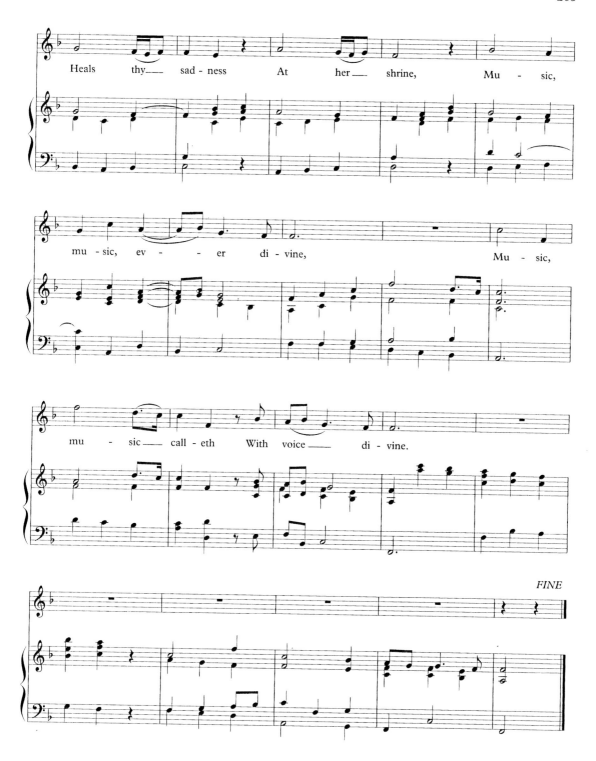

Heals thy___ sad - ness At her ___ shrine, Mu - sic,

mu - sic, ev - - er di - vine, Mu - sic,

mu - sic ___ call - eth With voice ___ di - vine.

FINE

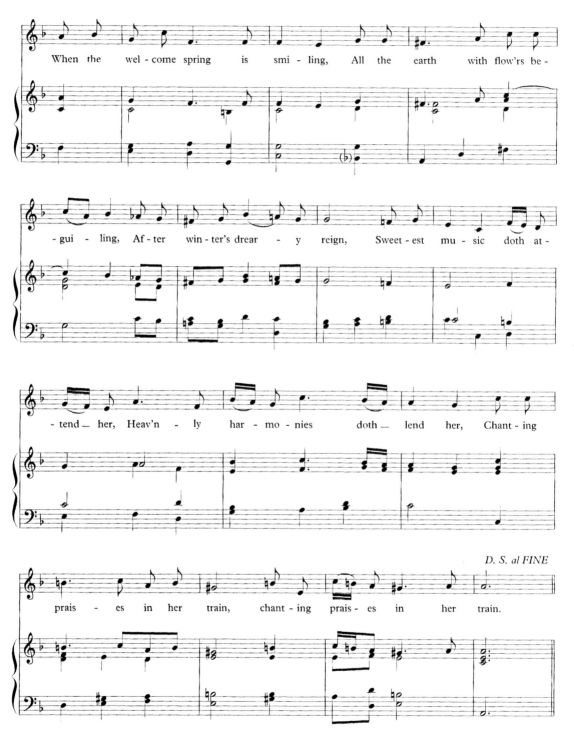

When the wel - come spring is smi - ling, All the earth with flow'rs be -
-gui - ling, Af - ter win - ter's drear — y reign, Sweet - est mu - sic doth at -
-tend — her, Heav'n - ly har - mo - nies doth — lend her, Chant - ing

D. S. al FINE

prais — es in her train, chant - ing prais - es in her train.

(Words by W. G. Rothery. Music by G. F. Handel.)

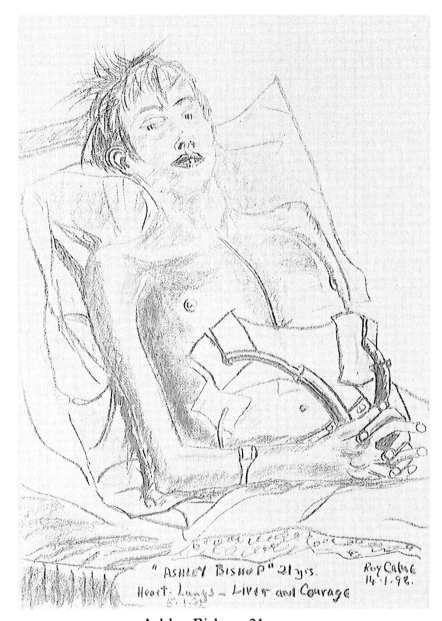

Ashley Bishop, 21 years.
'Heart Lungs Liver and Courage'. (14.1.92). *Roy Calne.*
This is a drawing by Sir Roy Calne of one of his patients recovering from an operation.

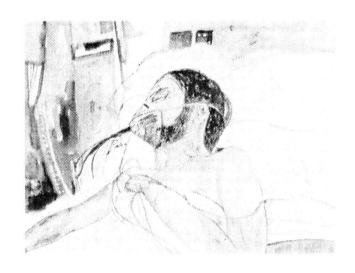

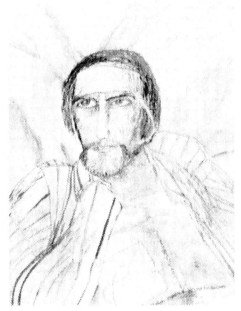

John Bellany, a major contemporary Scottish artist, received a liver transplant in Addenbrooke's hospital, Cambridge in 1988. The surgeon was Sir Roy Calne (see p. 205). As soon as he was out of the anaesthetic John Bellany asked for drawing material, and the creative energy involved in the self-portraits distracted him from the considerable pain he was in.

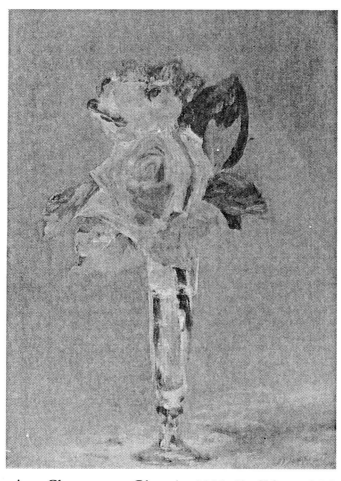

Roses in a Champagne Glass (c. 1881–3). *Edouard Manet.*
Manet's flower pictures were painted during the last two years of his life, in an order which cannot be known for certain. He had been ill for several years, probably of syphilis contracted in his earlier years. His illness accounts for the size of the paintings—this one is only 31 × 24 cm. Although there is a sadness about the paintings Manet, through his art, has overcome his disability and constant pain and invests the paintings with a sense of vitality. In painting the roses of this picture Manet must have remembered the two roses which stood in front of the beautiful barmaid in A Bar at the Folies-Bergere. *But there is no self-pity in the painting, despite the fact that he could work only in a seated position.*

Healing the Spirit

Richard Wagner
1813–1883

Biscuits as Therapy
From *a Letter to Mathilde Wesendonck*

Lucerne, 9 May 1859

CHILD, child! The biscuits did help; they suddenly jerked me out of a bad patch where I have been stuck for a week, unable to go further. Yesterday my attempts to work were miserably unsuccessful. I was in a shocking humour, and gave it vent in a long letter to Liszt in which I informed him that I had come to the end of my composing days. . . . Today I was staring up at the grey sky, utterly disconsolate, simply wondering to whom I could now write something acrimonious. For a whole week had gone by since I had made any progress in the actual composition; I was stuck at the transition from 'vor Sehnsucht nicht zu sterben' to Tristan's voyage (Act 3). So I had put that aside and turned back to work further on the beginning, the part I played to you. But today even that was making no progress, because I feel I did it much better before and cannot remember now how it was.

When the biscuits arrived, I realized what had been lacking; the biscuits I had here were much too salty, so they could not give me any sensible ideas; but when I took the sweet ones I had always been accustomed to, and dipped them in milk, everything suddenly fell into place. And so I threw aside the revision and went back to composing, on the story of the woman physician from far away. And now I am delighted; the transition is unbelievably successful, with a quite wonderful combination of two themes. Heavens, how much can be achieved by the right sort of biscuits!—Biscuits! that is the proper remedy for composers when they get stuck—but they must be the right kind. Now I have a good reserve of them; when you notice it getting low, be sure you send for more: I can see it is important . . .

(Translated from the German by Daphne Woodward)

Sidney Smith
1771–1845

Advice on Low Spirits
From *a Letter to Lady Georgiana Morpeth*

16 February 1820

NOBODY has suffered more from low spirits than I have done, so I feel for you. 1. Live as well and drink as much wine as you dare. 2. Go into the shower-bath with a small quantity of water at a temperature low enough to give you a *slight sensation of cold*—75 or 80°. 3. Amusing books. 4. Short views of human life not farther than dinner or tea. 5. Be as busy as you can. 6. See as much as you can of those friends who respect and like you; 7. and of those acquaintance who amuse you. 8. Make no secret of low spirits to your friends but talk of them fully: they are always the worse for dignified concealment. 9. Attend to the effects tea and coffee produce upon you. 10. Compare your lot with that of other people. 11. Don't expect too much of human life, a sorry business at the best. 12. Avoid poetry, dramatic representations (except comedy), music, serious novels, melancholy sentimental people, and everything likely to excite feeling or emotion not ending in active benevolence. 13. Do good and endeavour to please everybody of every degree. 14. Be as much as you can in the open air without fatigue. 15. Make the room where you commonly sit gay and pleasant. 16. Struggle by little and little against idleness. 17. Don't be too severe upon yourself, or underrate yourself, but do yourself justice. 18. Keep good blazing fires. 19. Be firm and constant in the exercise of rational religion. 20. Believe me dear Lady Georgiana very truly yours, Sydney Smith.

Alice Walker
1944–

Oppressed Hair Puts a Ceiling on the Brain

A FEW years ago I experienced one such long period of restlessness disguised as stillness. That is to say, I pretty much withdrew from the larger world in favor of the peace of my personal, smaller one. I unplugged myself from television and newspapers (a great relief!), from the more disturbing members of my extended family, and from most of my friends. I seemed to have reached a ceiling in my brain. And under this ceiling my mind was very restless, although all else about me was calm.

As one does in these periods of introspection, I counted the beads of my progress in this world. In my relationship to my family and the ancestors, I felt I had behaved respectfully (not all of them would agree, no doubt); in my work I felt I had done, to the best of my ability, all that was required of me; in my relationship to the persons with whom I daily shared my life I had acted with all the love I could possibly locate within myself. I was also at least beginning to acknowledge my huge responsibility to the Earth and my adoration of the Universe. What else, then, was required? Why was it that, when I meditated and sought the escape hatch at the top of my brain, which, at an earlier stage of growth, I had been fortunate enough to find, I now encountered a ceiling, as if the route to merge with the infinite I had become used to was plastered over?

One day, after I had asked this question earnestly for half a year, it occurred to me that in my physical self there remained one last barrier to my spiritual liberation, at least in the present phase: my hair.

Not my friend hair itself, for I quickly understood that it was innocent. It was the way I related to it that was the problem. I was always thinking about it. So much so that if my spirit had been a balloon eager to soar away and merge with the infinite, my hair would be the rock that anchored it to Earth. I realized that there was no hope of continuing my spiritual development, no hope of future growth of my soul, no hope of really being able to stare at the Universe and forget myself entirely in the staring (one of the purest joys!) if I still remained chained to thoughts about my hair. I suddenly understood why nuns and monks shaved their heads!

I looked at myself in the mirror and I laughed with happiness! I had broken through the seed skin, and was on my way upward through the earth.

Now I began to experiment: For several months I wore long braids (a fashion among black women at the time) made from the hair of Korean women. I loved this. It fulfilled my fantasy of having very long hair and it gave my short, mildly processed (oppressed) hair a chance to grow out. The young woman who braided my hair was someone I grew to love—a struggling young mother, she and her daughter would arrive at my house at seven in the evening and we would talk, listen to music, and eat pizza or burritos while she worked, until one or two o'clock in the morning. I loved the craft involved in the designs she created for my head.

(Basket making! a friend once cried on feeling the intricate weaving atop my head.) I loved sitting between her knees the way I used to sit between my mother's and sister's knees while they braided my hair when I was a child. I loved the fact that my own hair grew out and grew healthy under the 'extensions', as the lengths of hair were called. I loved paying a young sister for work that was truly original and very much a part of the black hair-styling tradition. I loved the fact that I did not have to deal with my hair except once every two or three months (for the first time in my life I could wash it every day if I wanted to and not have to do anything further). Still, eventually the braids would have to be taken down (a four-to-seven-hour job) and redone (another seven to eight hours); nor did I ever quite forget the Korean women, who, according to my young hairdresser, grew their hair expressly to be sold. Naturally this information caused me to wonder (and, yes, worry) about all other areas of their lives.

When my hair was four inches long, I dispensed with the hair of my Korean sisters and braided my own. It was only then that I became reacquainted with its natural character. I found it to be springy, soft, almost sensually responsive to moisture. As the little braids spun off in all directions but the ones I tried to encourage them to go, I discovered my hair's willfulness, so like my own! I saw that my friend hair, given its own life, had a sense of humor. I discovered I liked it.

(From *Living by the Word*, 1988)

George Herbert
1593–1633

Virtue

SWEET day, so cool, so calm, so bright,
The bridal of the earth and sky:
The dew shall weep thy fall tonight,
        For thou must die.

Sweet rose, whose hue angry and brave
Bids the rash gazer wipe his eye:
Thy root is ever in its grave,
        And thou must die.

Sweet spring, full of sweet days and roses,
A box where sweets compacted lie:
My music shows ye have your closes,
        And all must die.

Only a sweet and virtuous soul,
Like seasoned timber never gives;
But though the whole world turn to coal,
        Then chiefly lives.

Gerard Manley Hopkins
1844–1889

Peace

WHEN will you ever, Peace, wild wooddove, shy wings shut,
Your round me roaming end, and under be my boughs?
When, when, Peace, will you, Peace? I'll not play hypocrite
To own my heart: I yield you do come sometimes; but
That piecemeal peace is poor peace. What pure peace allows
Alarms of wars, the daunting wars, the death of it?

O surely, reaving Peace, my Lord should leave in lieu
Some good! And so he does leave Patience exquisite,
That plumes to Peace thereafter. And when Peace here does house
He comes with work to do, he does not come to coo,
        He comes to brood and sit.

Wilfred Owen
1893–1918

Hospital Barge at Cérisy

BUDGING the sluggard ripples of the Somme,
A barge round old Cérisy slowly slewed.
Softly her engines down the current screwed
And chuckled in her, with contented hum.
Till fairy tinklings struck their crooning dumb,
And waters rumpling at the stern subdued.
The lock-gate took her bulging amplitude.
Gently into the gurgling lock she swum.

One, reading by that sunset raised his eyes
To watch her lessening westward quietly;
Till, as she neared the bend, her funnel screamed.
And that long lamentation made him wise
How unto Avalon in agony
Kings passed in the dark barge which Merlin dreamed.

John Keats
1795–1821

To Sleep

O SOFT embalmer of the still midnight,
    Shutting with careful fingers and benign,
Our gloom-pleased eyes, embower'd from the light,
    Enshaded in forgetfulness divine:
O soothest Sleep! if so it please thee, close
    In midst of this thine hymn, my willing eyes,
Or wait the amen, ere thy poppy throws
    Around my bed its lulling charities.
    Then save me, or the passèd day will shine
Upon my pillow, breeding many woes;—
Save me from curious conscience, that still lords
    Its strength for darkness, burrowing like a mole;
Turn the key deftly in the oilèd wards,
    And seal the hushèd casket of my soul.

⇜6⇝
Last Things

*T*HE *themes of death, dying, and mourning have inspired the greatest art. There is so much material that it was convenient to organize it into three sections: attitudes to death, suffering and dying, funerals and mourning. The variety of attitudes and the range of feelings involved are a reflection of the inescapability of these events for us all. It must be noted, however, that our reactions to death are not always sad or despairing; humour of all kinds can be provoked by death. Indeed, that is one way in which the fear of death can be overcome. But the richness, the complexity, and the simplicity of the passages must be allowed to speak for themselves.*

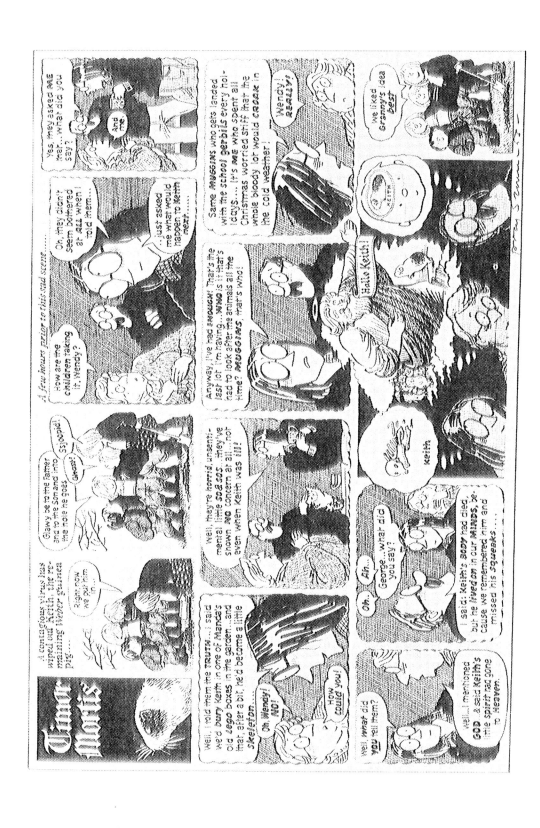

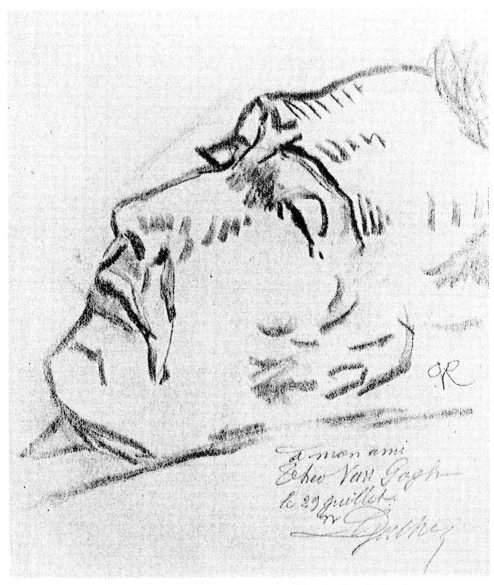

Vincent Van Gogh on His Deathbed. *Paul Gachet.*
Dr Paul Gachet was a friend to several Impressionist painters, and was himself a
competent painter. He was Van Gogh's doctor and had him to stay during
Van Gogh's last illness. Van Gogh painted Dr Gachet, and this drawing is by
Dr Gachet of Van Gogh on his deathbed in Auvers, 29 July 1890.

Attitudes to Death

Bible (Authorized Version)
From *Ecclesiastes (Ch. 12, vs 1–7)*

REMEMBER now thy Creator in the days of thy youth, while the evil days come not, nor the years draw nigh, when thou shalt say, I have no pleasure in them. While the sun, or the light, or the moon, or the stars, be not darkened, nor the clouds return after the rain: In the days when the keepers of the house shall tremble, and the strong men shall bow themselves, and the grinders cease because they are few, and those that look out of the windows be darkened, And the doors shall be shut in the streets, when the sound of the grinding is low, and he shall rise up at the voice of the bird, and all the daughters of musick shall be brought low; Also when they shall be afraid of that which is high, and fears shall be in the way, and the almond tree shall flourish, and the grasshopper shall be a burden, and desire shall fail: because man goeth to his long home, and the mourners go about the streets: Or ever the silver cord be loosed, or the golden bowl be broken, or the pitcher be broken at the fountain, or the wheel broken at the cistern. Then shall the dust return to the earth as it was: and the spirit shall return unto God who gave it.

Plato
c.428–c.348 BC
The Trial and Death of Socrates

[After the jury decided on the death-penalty, Socrates told them]

'DEATH is one of two things. Either it is annihilation, and the dead have no consciousness of anything; or, as we are told, it is really a change: a migration of the soul from this place to another. Now if there is no consciousness but only a dreamless sleep, death must be a marvellous gain. . . . If on the other hand, death is a removal from here to some other place, and if what we are told is true, that all the dead are there, what greater blessing could there be than this, gentlemen?' . . .

'You too, gentlemen of the jury, must look forward to death with confidence, and fix your minds on this one belief, which is certain: that nothing can harm a good man either in life or after death, and his fortunes are not a matter of indifference to the gods. This present experience of mine has not come about mechanically; I am quite clear that the time had come when it was better for me to die and be released from my distractions.'

[In prison, some time after drinking the poison]
Socrates walked about, and presently, saying that his legs were heavy, lay down on his back—that was what the man recommended. The man (he was the same one who had administered the poison) kept his hand upon Socrates, and after a little while examined his feet and legs; then pinched his foot hard and asked if he felt it. Socrates said no. Then he did the same to his legs; and moving gradually upwards in this way let us see that he was getting cold and numb. Presently he felt him again and said that when it reached the heart, Socrates would be gone.

The coldness was spreading about as far as his waist when Socrates uncovered his face—for he had covered it up—and said (these were his last words), 'Crito, we ought to offer a cock to Asclepius. See to it, and don't forget' *[to the god of health, after the sickness of life]*.

'No, it shall be done,' said Crito. 'Are you sure that there is nothing else?'

Socrates made no reply to this question, but after a little while he stirred; and when the man uncovered him, his eyes were fixed. When Crito saw this, he closed his mouth and eyes.

(From *Apology* and *Phaedo. Translated from the Greek by H. Tredennick*)

Sir Thomas Browne
1605–1682
From *Religio Medici*

WE terme sleepe a death, and yet it is waking that kils us, and destroyes those spirits which are the house of life. 'Tis indeed a part of life that best expresseth death, for every man truly lives so long as hee acts his nature, or someway makes good the faculties of himselfe: *Themistocles* therefore that slew his Souldier in his sleepe was a mercifull executioner; 'tis a kinde of punishment the mildness of no lawes hath invented; I wonder the fancy of *Lucan* and *Seneca* did not discover it. It is that death by which we may be literally said to die daily, a death which *Adam* died before his mortality; a death whereby we live a middle and moderating point between life and death; in fine, so like death, I dare not trust it without my prayers, and so halfe adiew unto the world, and take my farewell in a Colloquy with God.

John Donne
1572–1631

From *Holy Sonnets*

DEATH, be not proud, though some have called thee
Mighty and dreadful, for thou art not so;
For those whom thou thinkst thou dost overthrow
Die not, poor Death, nor yet canst thou kill me.
From rest and sleep, which but thy pictures be,
Much pleasure—then, from thee much more must flow;
And soonest our best men with thee do go,
Rest of their bones and soul's delivery.
Thou'rt slave to fate, chance, kings, and desperate men,
And dost with poison, war, and sickness dwell;
And poppy or charms can make us sleep as well,
And better than thy stroke. Why swellst thou then?
One short sleep past, we wake eternally,
And death shall be no more. Death, thou shalt die.

John Keats
1795–1821

When I Have Fears that I May Cease to Be

WHEN I have fears that I may cease to be
Before my pen has glean'd my teeming brain,
Before high-pilèd books, in charact'ry,
Hold like rich garners the full-ripen'd grain;
When I behold, upon the night's starr'd face,
Huge cloudy symbols of a high romance,
And feel that I may never live to trace
Their shadows, with the magic hand of chance;
And when I feel, fair creature of an hour!
That I shall never look upon thee more,
Never have relish in the faery power
Of unreflecting love;—then on the shore
  Of the wide world I stand alone, and think,
  Till Love and Fame to nothingness do sink.

Wilfred Owen
1893–1918

Futility

MOVE him into the sun—
Gently its touch awoke him once,
At home, whispering of fields half-sown.
Always it woke him, even in France,
Until this morning and this snow.
If anything might rouse him now
The kind old sun will know.

Think how it wakes the seeds—
Woke once the clays of a cold star.
Are limbs, so dear achieved, are sides
Full-nerved, still warm, too hard to stir?
Was it for this the clay grew tall?
—O what made fatuous sunbeams toil
To break earth's sleep at all?

Robert Bly
1926–

Counting Small-Boned Bodies

LET'S count the bodies over again.

If we could only make the bodies smaller,
the size of skulls,
we could make a whole plain white with skulls in the
    moonlight.

If we could only make the bodies smaller,
maybe we could fit
a whole year's kill in front of us on a desk.

If we could only make the bodies smaller,
we could fit
a body into a finger ring, for a keepsake forever.

[*Editor's Note:* This is an anti-Vietnam poem, but
splendid in its irony and sarcasm against *counting*
deaths]

Lenrie Peters
1932–

Watching Someone Die

WATCHING someone die
is a fraudulent experience
The deep significance is felt
the meaning escapes
like a child's first punishment.
The dying ravish your strength
whether by throttle of convulsive gasp
or tideless fading away
like ancient familiar sounds in sea shells
the moment is the same
reinforced brutality to life
a rugged cliff bloodstained
with the agonising rhythm of many heads.
A cold demise; each
successive moment a banishment.
The terror is in leaving behind
the ache is in departing.

Humming fantasies crowd their stings
to seize and record the moment
the hands curl in spasm
to hold it back; this life, this infidel.
It is too late. Everything and nothing
has happened. A huge machine
the earth, grinds to a bolt-knocking halt.

It is the changing of the tide
at the boundary hour
Life like a handful of feathers
engulfed by cliff winds
one like yourself swept

Oh so swiftly into the anchorage of history
Tears and sighs; sighs and tears
stamping the leaden feet
the solid agony of years
they all abound.
One life or a million
contrived by nature or by man
greatly obscures the issue.

Face to face with dying
you are none-the-wiser
Yet it seems a most ignoble epitaph
'He was a man and had to die; after all.'

George Meredith
1828–1909

A Wind Sways the Pines

A WIND sways the pines,
And below
Not a breath of wild air;
Still as the mosses that glow
On the flooring and over the lines
Of the roots here and there.
The pine tree drops its dead;
They are quiet, as under the sea.
Overhead, overhead
Rushes life in a race,
As the clouds the clouds chase;
  And we go,
And we drop like the fruits of the tree,
    Even we,
    Even so.

A. E. Housman
1859–1936

From *A Shropshire Lad*

FROM far, from eve and morning
   And yon twelve-winded sky,
The stuff of life to knit me
   Blew hither: here am I.

Now—for a breath I tarry
   Nor yet disperse apart—
Take my hand quick and tell me,
   What have you in your heart.

Speak now, and I will answer;
   How shall I help you, say;
Ere to the wind's twelve quarters
   I take my endless way.

Edwin Muir
1887–1959

The Child Dying

UNFRIENDLY friendly universe,
I pack your stars into my purse,
And bid you, bid you so farewell.
That I can leave you, quite go out,
Go out, go out beyond all doubt,
My father says, is the miracle.

You are so great, and I so small:
I am nothing, you are all:
Being nothing, I can take this way.
Oh I need neither rise nor fall,
For when I do not move at all
I shall be out of all your day.

It's said some memory will remain
In the other place, grass in the rain,
Light on the land, sun on the sea,
A flitting grace, a phantom face,
But the world is out. There is no place
Where it and its ghost can ever be.

Father, father, I dread this air
Blown from the far side of despair,
The cold cold corner. What house, what hold,
What hand is there? I look and see
Nothing-filled eternity,
And the great round world grows weak and old.

Hold my hand, oh hold it fast—
I am changing!—until at last
My hand in yours no more will change,
Though yours change on. You here, I there,
So hand in hand, twin-leafed despair—
I did not know death was so strange.

Norman Maclean
1902–1990

From *A River Runs through It*

WE sat on the bank and the river went by. As always, it was making sounds to itself, and now it made sounds to us. It would be hard to find three men sitting side by side who knew better what a river was saying.

On the Big Blackfoot River above the mouth of Belmont Creek the banks are fringed by large Ponderosa pines. In the slanting sun of late afternoon the shadows of great branches reached from across the river, and the trees took the river in their arms. The shadows continued up the bank, until they included us.

A river, though, has so many things to say that it is hard to know what it says to each of us. As we were packing our tackle and fish in the car, Paul repeated, 'Just give me three more years.' At the time, I was surprised at the repetition, but later I realized that the river somewhere, sometime, must have told me, too, that he would receive no such gift. For, when the police sergeant early next May wakened me before daybreak, I rose and asked no questions. Together we drove across the Continental Divide and down the length of the Big Blackfoot River over forest floors yellow and sometimes white with glacier lilies to tell my father and mother that my brother had been beaten to death by the butt of a revolver and his body dumped in an alley.

My mother turned and went to her bedroom where, in a house full of men and rods and rifles, she had faced most of her great problems alone. She was never to ask me a question about the man she loved most and understood least. Perhaps she knew enough to know that for her it was enough to have loved him. He was probably the only man in the world who had held her in his arms and leaned back and laughed.

When I finished talking to my father, he asked, 'Is there anything else you can tell me?'

Finally, I said, 'Nearly all the bones in his hand were broken.'

He almost reached the door and then turned back for reassurance. 'Are you sure that the bones in his hand were broken?' he asked. I repeated, 'Nearly all the bones in his hand were broken.' 'In which hand?' he asked. 'In his right hand,' I answered.

After my brother's death, my father never walked very well again. He had to struggle to lift his feet, and, when he did get them up, they came down slightly out of control. From time to time Paul's right hand had to be reaffirmed; then my father would shuffle away again. He could not shuffle in a straight line from trying to lift his feet. Like many Scottish ministers before him, he had to derive what comfort he could from the faith that his son had died fighting.

For some time, though, he struggled for more to hold on to. 'Are you sure you have told me everything you know about his death?' he asked. I said, 'Everything.' 'It's not much, is it?' 'No,' I replied, 'but you can love completely without complete understanding.' 'That I have known and preached,' my father said.

Once my father came back with another question. 'Do you think I could have helped him?' he asked. Even if I might have thought longer, I would have made the same answer. 'Do you think I could have helped him?' I answered. We stood waiting in deference to each other. How can a question be answered that asks a lifetime of questions?

After a long time he came with something he must have wanted to ask from the first. 'Do you think it was just a stick-up and foolishly he tried to fight his way out? You know what I mean—that it wasn't connected with anything in his past.'

'The police don't know,' I said.

'But do you?' he asked, and I felt the implication.

'I've said I've told you all I know. If you push me far enough, all I really know is that he was a fine fisherman.'

'You know more than that,' my father said. 'He was beautiful.'

'Yes,' I said, 'he was beautiful. He should have been—you taught him.'

My father looked at me for a long time—he just looked at me. So this was the last he and I ever said to each other about Paul's death.

Indirectly, though, he was present in many of our conversations. Once, for instance, my father asked me a series of questions that suddenly made me wonder whether I understood even my father whom I felt closer to than any man I have ever known. 'You like to tell true stories, don't you?' he asked, and I answered, 'Yes, I like to tell stories that are true.'

Then he asked, 'After you have finished your true stories sometime, why don't you make up a story and the people to go with it?

'Only then will you understand what happened and why.

'It is those we live with and love and should know who elude us.'

Now nearly all those I loved and did not understand when I was young are dead, but I still reach out to them.

Of course, now I am too old to be much of a fisherman, and now of course I usually fish the big waters alone, although some friends think I shouldn't. Like many fly fishermen in western Montana where the summer days are almost Arctic in length, I often do not start fishing until the cool of the evening. Then in the Arctic half-light of the canyon, all existence fades to a being with my soul and memories and the sounds of the Big Blackfoot River and a four-count rhythm and the hope that a fish will rise.

Eventually, all things merge into one, and a river runs through it. The river was cut by the world's great flood and runs over rocks from the basement of time. On some of the rocks are timeless raindrops. Under the rocks are the words, and some of the words are theirs.

I am haunted by waters.

(1976)

Thomas Campion
1567–1620

Never Weather-Beaten Saile

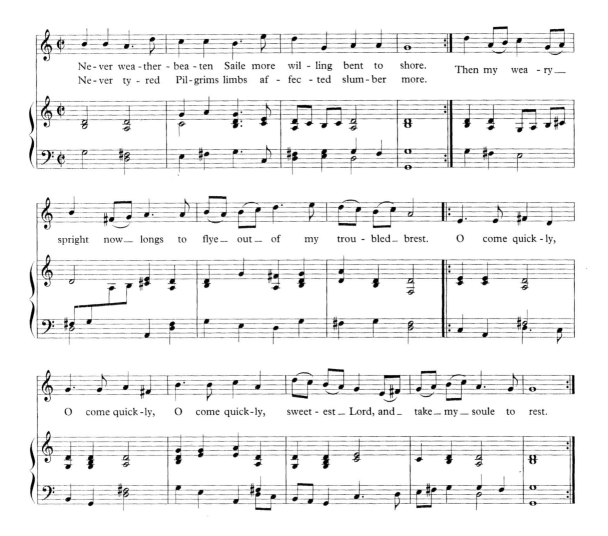

Ne-ver wea-ther-bea-ten Saile more wil-ling bent to shore.
Ne-ver ty-red Pil-grims limbs af-fec-ted slum-ber more. Then my wea-ry

spright now— longs to flye— out— of my trou-bled— brest. O come quick-ly,

O come quick-ly, O come quick-ly, sweet-est— Lord, and— take— my— soule to rest.

Ever-blooming are the joyes of Heav'ns high paradice,
Cold age deafes not there our eares, nor vapour dims our eyes;
Glory there the Sun outshines, whose beames the blessed onely see:
O come quickly, glorious Lord, and raise my spright to thee.

✦ Suffering and Dying

W. H. Auden
1907–1973

Musée des Beaux Arts

ABOUT suffering they were never wrong,
The Old Masters: how well they understood
Its human position; how it takes place
While someone else is eating or opening a window or just walking dully along;
How, when the aged are reverently, passionately waiting
For the miraculous birth, there always must be
Children who did not specially want it to happen, skating
On a pond at the edge of the wood:
They never forgot
That even the dreadful martyrdom must run its course
Anyhow in a corner, some untidy spot
Where the dogs go on with their doggy life and the torturer's horse
Scratches its innocent behind on a tree.

In Brueghel's *Icarus*, for instance: how everything turns away
Quite leisurely from the disaster; the ploughman may
Have heard the splash, the forsaken cry,
But for him it was not an important failure; the sun shone
As it had to on the white legs disappearing into the green
Water; and the expensive delicate ship that must have seen
Something amazing, a boy falling out of the sky,
Had somewhere to get to and sailed calmly on.

John Stone
1936–

Death

I HAVE seen   come on
slowly as rust
sand

or suddenly   as when
someone leaving
a room

finds the doorknob
come loose in his hand

Philip Larkin
1922–1985

Cut Grass

CUT grass lies frail:
Brief is the breath
Mown stalks exhale.
Long, long the death

It dies in the white hours
Of young-leafed June
With chestnut flowers,
With hedges snowlike strewn,

White lilac bowed,
Lost lanes of Queen Anne's lace,
And that high-builded cloud
Moving at summer's pace.

Simone de Beauvoir
1908–1986

From *A Very Easy Death*

AT 9 o'clock [Dr] N came out of the room and said angrily, 'Another clip has given way. After all that has been done for her: how irritating!' He went off, leaving my sister dumbfounded. In spite of her icy hands Maman complained of being too hot, and she had some difficulty in breathing. She was given an injection and she went to sleep. Poupette undressed, got into bed and went through the motions of reading a detective story. Towards midnight Maman moved about. Poupette and the nurse went to her bedside. She opened her eyes. 'What are you doing here? Why are you looking so worried? I am quite well.' 'You have been having a bad dream.' As Mademoiselle Cournot smoothed the sheets she touched Maman's feet: there was the chill of death upon them. My sister wondered whether to call me. But at that time of night my presence would have frightened Maman, whose mind was perfectly clear. Poupette went back to bed. At 1 o'clock Maman stirred again. In a roguish voice she whispered the words of an old refrain that Papa used to sing, *You are going away and you will leave us.* 'No, no,' said Poupette, 'I shan't leave you,' and Maman gave a little knowing smile. She found it harder and harder to breathe. After another injection she murmured in a rather thick voice, 'We must . . . keep . . . back . . . desh.'

'We must keep back the desk?'

'No,' said Maman. 'Death.' Stressing the word *death* very strongly. She added, 'I don't want to die.'

'But you are better now!'

After that she wandered a little. 'I should have liked to have the time to bring out my book. . . . She must be allowed to nurse whoever she likes.'

My sister dressed herself: Maman had almost lost consciousness. Suddenly she cried, 'I can't breathe!' Her mouth opened, her eyes stared wide, huge in that wasted, ravaged face: with a spasm she entered into coma.

'Go and telephone,' said Mademoiselle Cournot.

Poupette rang me up: I did not answer. The operator went on ringing for half an hour before I woke. Meanwhile Poupette went back to Maman: already she was no longer there—her heart was beating and she breathed, sitting there with glassy eyes that saw nothing. And then it was over. 'The doctors said she would go out like a candle: it wasn't like that, it wasn't like that at all,' said my sister, sobbing.

'But, Madame,' replied the nurse, 'I assure you it was a very easy death.'

(Translated from the French by P. O'Brian)

J. E. Austen-Leigh
1798–1874

From *Memoir of Jane Austen*

THROUGHOUT her illness she was nursed by her sister, often assisted by her sister-in-law, my mother. Both were with her when she died. Two of her brothers, who were clergymen, lived near enough to Winchester to be in frequent attendance, and to administer the services suitable for a Christian's death-bed. While she used the language of hope to her correspondents, she was fully aware of her danger, though not appalled by it. It is true that there was much to attach her to life. She was happy in her family; she was just beginning to feel confidence in her own success; and, no doubt, the exercise of her great talents was an enjoyment in itself. We may well believe that she would gladly have lived longer; but she was enabled without dismay or complaint to prepare for death. She was a humble, believing Christian. Her life had been passed in the performance of home duties and the cultivation of domestic affections, without any self-seeking or craving after applause. She had always sought, as it were by instinct, to promote the happiness of all who came within her influence, and doubtless she had her reward in the peace of mind which was granted to her in her last days. Her sweetness of temper never failed. She was ever considerate and grateful to those who attended on her. At times, when she felt rather better, her playfulness of spirit revived, and she amused them even in her sadness. Once, when she thought herself near her end, she said what she imagined might be her last words to those around her, and particularly thanked her sister-in-law for being with her, saying, 'You have always been a kind sister to me, Mary.' When the end at last came, she sank rapidly, and on being asked by her attendants whether there was anything that she wanted, her reply was, 'Nothing but death.' These were her last words. In quietness and peace she breathed her last on the morning of 18 July 1817.

Matthew Arnold
1822–1888

From *A Wish*

SPARE me the whispering, crowded room,
The friends who come, and gape, and go;
The ceremonious air of gloom—
All, that makes death a hideous show!

Nor bring, to see me cease to live,
Some doctor full of phrase and fame,
To shake his sapient head and give
The ill he cannot cure a name.

Nor fetch, to take the accustom'd toll
Of the poor sinner bound for death,
His brother doctor of the soul,
To canvass with official breath

The future and its viewless things—
That undiscover'd mystery
Which one who feels death's winnowing wings
Must needs read clearer, sure, than he!

Bring none of these! but let me be,
While all around in silence lies,
Moved to the window near, and see
Once more before my dying eyes

Bathed in the sacred dews of morn
The wide aërial landscape spread—
The world which was ere I was born,
The world which lasts when I am dead.

Florence Nightingale
1820–1910

From *Notes on Nursing*

I REALLY believe there is scarcely a greater worry which invalids have to endure than the incurable hopes of their friends . . . attempting to 'cheer' the sick by making light of their danger and by exaggerating their probabilities of recovery. . . . The fact is, that the patient is not 'cheered' at all by these well-meaning, most tiresome friends. On the contrary, he is depressed and wearied. If, on the one hand, he exerts himself to tell each successive member of this too numerous conspiracy, whose name is legion, why he does not think as they do,—in what respect he is worse,—what symptoms exist that they know nothing of,—he is fatigued instead of 'cheered', and his attention is fixed upon himself. In general, patients who are really ill, do not want to talk about themselves . . .

If, on the other hand, and which is much more frequently the case, the patient says nothing, but the Shakespearian 'Oh!' 'Ah!' 'Go to!' and 'In good sooth!' in order to escape from the conversation about himself the sooner, he is depressed by want of sympathy. He feels isolated in the midst of friends. He feels what a convenience it would be, if there were any single person to whom he could speak simply and openly, without pulling the string upon himself of this shower-bath of silly hopes and encouragements; to whom he could express his wishes and directions without that person persisting in saying, 'I hope that it will please God yet to give you twenty years,' or, 'You have a long life of activity before you.' How often we see at the end of biographies or of cases recorded in medical papers, 'after a long illness A. died rather suddenly,' or, 'unexpectedly both to himself and to others'. 'Unexpectedly' to others, perhaps, who did not see, because they did not look; but by no means 'unexpectedly to himself', as I feel entitled to believe, both from the internal evidence in such stories, and from watching similar cases; there was every reason to expect that A. would die, and he knew it; but he found it useless to insist upon his own knowledge to his friends. . . .

Charles Dickens
1812–1870

From *Bleak House*

AFTER watching him closely a little while, Allan puts his mouth very near his ear, and says to him in a low, distinct voice:

'Jo! Did you every know a prayer?'

'Never knowd nothink, sir'

'Never so much as one short prayer?'

'No, sir. Nothink at all. Mr Chadbands he wos a-praying wunst at Mr Sangsby's and I heerd him, but he sounded as if he wos a-speakin' to hisself, and not to me. He prayed a lot, but *I* couldn't make out nothink on it. Different times, there was other genlmen come down Tom-all-Alone's a-praying, but they all mostly sed as the t'other wuns prayed wrong, and all mostly sounded to be a-talking to theirselves, or a-passing blame on the t'others, and not a-talkin to us. *We* never knowd nothink. *I* never knowd what it wos all about.'

It takes him a long time to say this; and few but an experienced and attentive listener could hear, or, hearing, understand him. After a short relapse into sleep or stupor, he makes, of a sudden, a strong effort to get out of bed.

'Stay Jo! What now?'

'It's time for me to go to that there berryin ground, sir,' he returns with a wild look.

'Lie down, and tell me. What burying ground, Jo?'

'Where they laid him as wos wery good to me, wery good to me indeed, he wos. It's time fur me to go down to that there berryin ground, sir, and ask to be put along with him. I wants to go there and be berried. He used fur to say to me, 'I am as poor as you today, Jo,' he ses. I wants to tell him that I am as poor as him now, and have come there to be laid along with him.'

'By-and-by, Jo. By-and-by.'

'Ah! P'raps they wouldn't do it if I wos to go myself. But will you promise to have me took there, sir, and laid along with him?'

'I will, indeed.'

'Thank'ee sir. Thank'ee, sir. They'll have to get the key of the gate afore they can take me in, for it's allus locked. And there's a step there, as I used fur to clean with my broom.—It's turned wery dark, sir. Is there any light a-comin?'

'It is coming fast, Jo.'

Fast. The cart is shaken all to pieces, and the rugged road is very near its end.

'Jo, my poor fellow!'

'I hear you, sir, in the dark, but I'm a-gropin—a-gropin—let me catch hold of your hand.'

'Jo, can you say what I say?'

'I'll say anythink as you say, sir, for I knows it's good.'

'OUR FATHER.'

'Our Father!'—'yes, that's wery good sir.'

'WHICH ART IN HEAVEN.'

'Art in Heaven—is the light a-comin, sir?'

'It is close at hand. HALLOWED BE THY NAME!'

'Hallowed be—thy –'

The light is come upon the dark benighted way. Dead!

Dead, your Majesty. Dead, my lords and gentlemen. Dead, Right Reverends and Wrong Reverends of every order. Dead, men and women, born with Heavenly compassion in your hearts. And dying thus around us every day.

Douglas Dunn
1942–

France

A DOZEN sparrows scuttled on the frost.
We watched them play. We stood at the window,
And, if you saw us, then you saw a ghost
In duplicate. I tied her nightgown's bow.
She watched and recognized the passers-by.
Had they looked up, they'd know that she was ill—
'Please, do not draw the curtains when I die'—
From all the flowers on the windowsill.

'It's such a shame,' she said. 'Too ill, too quick.'
'I would have liked us to have gone away.'
We closed our eyes together, dreaming France,
Its meadows, rivers, woods and jouissance,
I counted summers, our love's arithmetic.
'Some other day, my love. Some other day.'

E. M. Forster
1879–1970

From *Howard's End*

IT was not unexpected entirely. Aunt Juley's health had been bad all the winter. She had had a long series of colds and coughs, and had been too busy to get rid of them. She had scarcely promised her niece 'to really take my tiresome chest in hand,' when she caught a chill and developed acute pneumonia. Margaret and Tibby went down to Swanage. Helen was telegraphed for, and that spring party that after all gathered in that hospitable house had all the pathos of fair memories. On a perfect day, when the sky seemed blue porcelain, and the waves of the discreet little bay beat the gentlest of tattoos upon the sand, Margaret hurried up through the rhododendrons, confronted again by the senselessness of Death. One death may explain itself, but it throws no light upon another: the groping inquiry must begin anew. Preachers or scientists may generalize, but we know that no generality is possible about those whom we love; not one heaven awaits them, not even one oblivion. Aunt Juley, incapable of tragedy, slipped out of life with odd little laughs and apologies for having stopped in it so long. She was very weak; she could not rise to the occasion, or realize the great mystery which all agree must await her; it only seemed to her that she was quite done up—more done up than ever before; that she saw and heard and felt less every moment; and that, unless something changed, she would soon feel nothing. Her spare strength she devoted to plans: could not Margaret take some steamer expeditions? were mackerel cooked as Tibby liked them? She worried herself about Helen's absence, and also that she should be the cause of Helen's return. The nurses seemed to think such interests quite natural, and perhaps hers was an average approach to the Great Gate. But Margaret saw Death stripped of any false romance; whatever the idea of Death may contain, the process can be trivial and hideous.

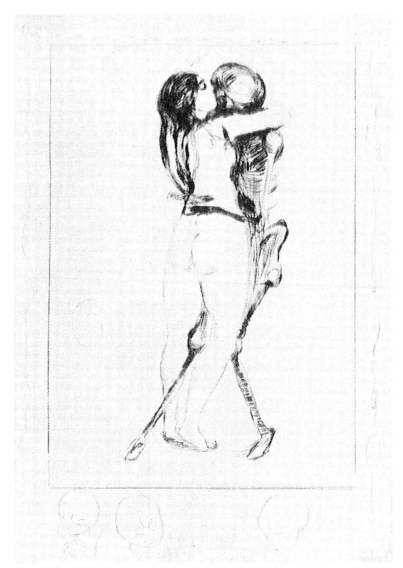

The Maiden and Death (1894). *Edvard Munch.*
Edvard Munch (1863–1944) was the son of a doctor in the poor quarter of Oslo. While he was still very young his mother and one sister died of consumption, and another sister died after becoming mentally deranged. It is therefore not surprising that themes of death and madness pervade his work. In this drawing the maiden is by no means reluctant to embrace death and seems to be welcoming him with a passionate kiss. In Schubert's song, by contrast, the maiden is afraid of death, who is described in the words and music as gentle and reassuring.

Franz Schubert
1797–1828

Der Tod und das Mädchen
(Death and the Maiden)

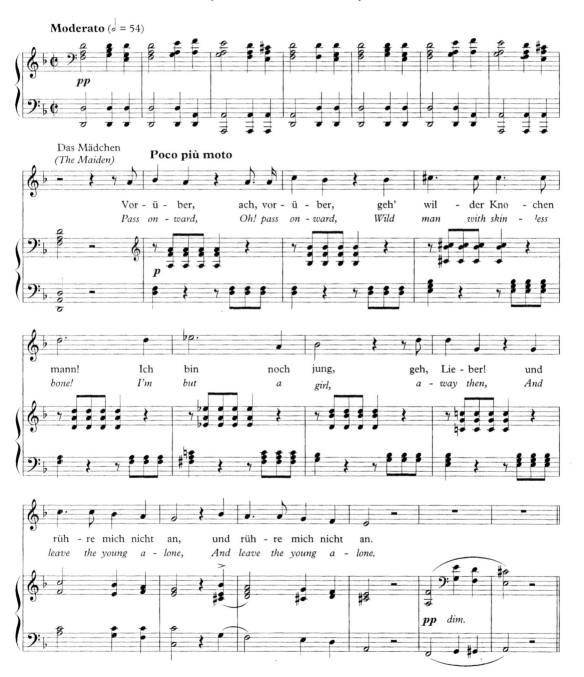

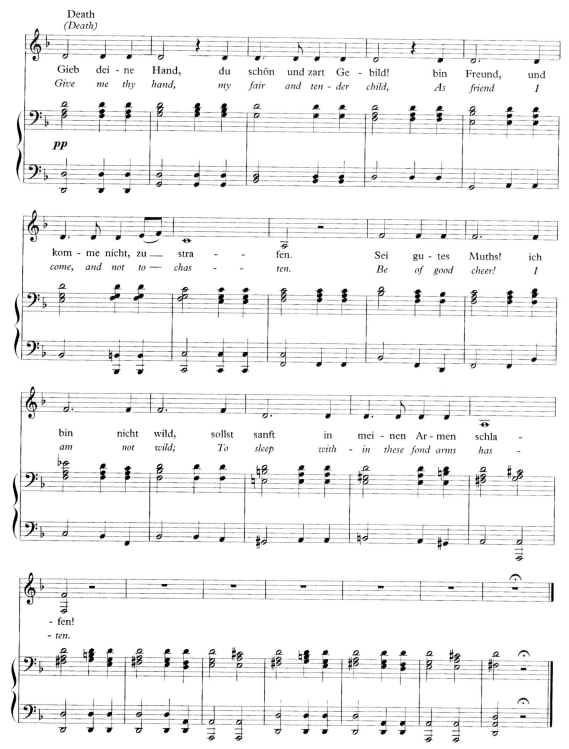

Death
(Death)

Gieb dei - ne Hand,   du schön und zart Ge - bild!   bin Freund,   und
Give   me   thy   hand,   my   fair   and ten - der child,   As   friend   I

kom - me nicht, zu __ stra - - fen.   Sei gu - tes Muths!   ich
come, and not to — chas - - ten.   Be   of good cheer!   I

bin   nicht wild,   sollst sanft   in   mei - nen Ar - men schla -
am   not   wild;   To   sleep   with - in   these fond arms   has -

- fen!
- ten.

German lyric: Matthias Claudius 1740–1815
English translation: Theodore Baker

Mourning and Funerals

John Davies of Hereford
1565–1618

A Remembrance of My Friend Mr Thomas Morley
DEATH hath deprived me of my dearest friend,
My dearest friend is dead and laid in grave,
In grave he rests until the world shall end,
The world shall end as end must all things have.
All things must have an end that nature wrought,
That nature wrought must unto dust be brought.

Seamus Heaney
1939–

Mid-Term Break
I SAT all morning in the college sick bay
Counting bells knelling classes to a close.
At two o'clock our neighbours drove me home.

In the porch I met my father crying –
He had always taken funerals in his stride –
And Big Jim Evans saying it was a hard blow.

The baby cooed and laughed and rocked the pram
When I came in, and I was embarrassed
By old men standing up to shake my hand

And tell me they were 'sorry for my trouble'.
Whispers informed strangers I was the eldest,
Away at school, as my mother held my hand

In hers and coughed out angry tearless sighs.
At ten o'clock the ambulance arrived
With the corpse, stanched and bandaged by the nurses.

Next morning I went up into the room. Snowdrops
And candles soothed the bedside; I saw him
For the first time in six weeks. Paler now,

Wearing a poppy bruise on his left temple,
He lay in the four foot box as in his cot.
No gaudy scars, the bumper knocked him clear.

A four foot box, a foot for every year.

George Mackay Brown
1921–

Shroud

SEVEN threads make the shroud,
The white thread,
A green corn thread,
A blue fish thread,
A red stitch, rut and rieving and wrath,
A gray thread
(All winter failing hand falleth on wheel)
The black thread,
And a thread too bright for the eye.

William Carlos Williams
1883–1963

Tract

I WILL teach you my townspeople
how to perform a funeral
for you have it over a troop
of artists—
unless one should scour the world—
you have the ground sense necessary.

See! the hearse leads.
I begin with a design for a hearse.
For Christ's sake not black—
nor white either—and not polished!
Let it be weathered—like a farm wagon—
with gilt wheels (this could be
applied fresh at small expense)
or no wheels at all:
a rough dray to drag over the ground.

Knock the glass out!
My God—glass, my townspeople!
For what purpose? Is it for the dead
to look out or for us to see
how well he is housed or to see
the flowers or the lack of them—
or what?
To keep the rain and snow from him?
He will have a heavier rain soon:
pebbles and dirt and what not.
Let there be no glass—
and no upholstery, phew!
and no little brass rollers
and small easy wheels on the bottom—
my townspeople what are you thinking of?

A rough plain hearse then
with gilt wheels and no top at all.
On this the coffin lies
by its own weight.

No wreaths please—
especially no hot house flowers.
Some common memento is better,
something he prized and is known by:
his old clothes—a few books perhaps –
God knows what! You realize
how we are about these things
my townspeople—
something will be found—anything
even flowers if he had come to that.
So much for the hearse.

For heaven's sake though see to the driver!
Take off the silk hat! In fact
that's no place at all for him—
up there unceremoniously
dragging our friend out to his own dignity!
Bring him down—bring him down!
Low and inconspicuous! I'd not have him ride
on the wagon at all—damn him—
the undertaker's understrapper!
Let him hold the reins
and walk at the side
and inconspicuously too!

Then briefly as to yourselves:
Walk behind—as they do in France,
seventh class, or if you ride
Hell take curtains! Go with some show
of inconvenience; sit openly—
to the weather as to grief.

Or do you think you can shut grief in?
What—from us? We who have perhaps nothing to lose? Share with us
share with us—it will be money
in your pockets.
Go now
I think you are ready.

Penelope Lively
1933–

From *Passing On*

THE coffin stuck fast at the angle of the garden path and the gateway out into the
road. The undertaker's men shunted to and fro, their hats knocked askew by low
branches, their topcoats showered with raindrops from the hedge. The mourners
halted around the front door and waited in silence. Birds sang effusively. At last
the men managed to pivot the coffin on the gatepost and proceeded to the waiting
hearse. The coffin was loaded. The mourners straggled out into the road and
hesitated, unwilling to commit themselves to the attendant limousines.

Louise said, 'It's daft using cars to go such a short distance. At least we could
have squashed into one, surely?'

There were two Daimlers. Helen and Edward got into the first, the four Dysons
into the second. First time I've ever ridden in one of these, thought Helen. The last
too, let's hope. They moved off at walking pace, past the Britches, radiant still with
birdsong, past the builders' yard where Ron Paget, heaving planks of timber from
the pick-up, suspended the operation and stood in respect, his eyes lowered. Helen
nudged Edward: 'The old rogue—look at him.' Edward nodded. He said, 'At least
he's not coming to the church—I wouldn't have put it past him.' Now they were
passing the shop, where the Birds Eye van driver continued to lift out cartons
without looking up. From within, faces watched furtively. Two women with
prams paused, tucking themselves into the wall as the cortège went by. A small
child pointed, questioning. They are having to explain, Helen thought. About
deaths, funerals. Probably they will dodge the issue with distractions—an iced
lollie, a sweetie. All the same, mother has disrupted the lives of others, just a little,
for the last time.

Now they were at the church, unloading. The coffin, the flowers, the mourners.

Through the lych gate, along the path, a halt at the door to make adjustments before entering. Two of the undertaker's men were young, Helen noticed; what a very curious choice of occupation. Earlier, she had looked out of the window at Greystones and seen one of them filling in a football coupon while they waited in the hearse. Now, their faces were composed into expressions of noncommittal sobriety.

'You three should go in first,' said Tim Dyson. 'I'll follow with the children.'

Only two of the family wore black. Tim's suit was a dark pinstripe but Edward's was green, shiny around the seat and elbows, brought out for school speech days and probably twenty years old. Helen had put on her camel coat; the late May morning was quite cold and she felt the coat to be more subdued than her maroon suit, the only other garment suitable for a formal occasion. Louise was in a hotchpotch of unashamed colour and pattern. The two adolescents, alone, were appropriately funereal, clad from head to toe in black leather.

There were twenty or thirty people in the church. The front pew had been left empty. The family shuffled into it. Helen, between her brother and sister, observed the coffin, which had been placed in the aisle just below the steps to the chancel.

It seemed, now, much too small. Helen thought of her mother's stocky form, eyed the coffin, and could not imagine her squeezed into it. She gazed at the varnished wood and the brass handles and waited to hear cries of protest and complaint. She half expected to have to rise to her feet and set things right. Glancing at Edward, she knew that he was thinking exactly the same.

'Let us pray. . . .'

Helen sank obediently to her knees. She said, O God, now that she is Thine rather than mine, do something about her. If she was created in Thy Image, then the system is an imperfect one.

'We consume away in Thy displeasure: and are afraid at Thy wrathful indignation. . . .'

No, not mother. She wasn't much more of a Christian than I am. A token one, being a natural conservative. But I doubt if she ever gave a thought to Thy displeasure, any more than to anyone else's.

The service proceeded. The congregation sang a hymn, creakily. Louise and the children were silent; Edward and Helen moved their lips; Tim Dyson gave tongue firmly in a light tenor. Helen allowed herself a glance sideways and backwards to see who was there. Expected faces. Village faces, more distant relatives, Doctor Taylor, someone middle-aged who must be Mr Carnaby from Carnaby and

Proctor, solicitors, to whom Helen had spoken on the phone but had not met. Dorothy Glover, at 80, had not had friends. Indeed she had not had many at 60 or at 40 or even, perhaps, at 20. Helen could think only of someone she did voluntary nursing with during the war, who sent Christmas cards, and a woman who shared her interest in a mystical form of healing involving a black box with a lot of wires and buttons, with whom she corresponded.

Mother was not a nice woman; I have always known that, and I can say it, because I am her daughter and so in the nature of things came nearer to loving her than anyone else ever did. As did Edward. Louise's attitude is rather different, for various reasons.

Louise, right now, appeared to be suffering. Her face had become contorted; she was reaching for a Kleenex with which she scrubbed both eyes, angrily. As the hymn ground to its end she hissed to Helen, 'Bloody hay fever! It's those blasted flowers. Why did we have to have them?'

'Because they were sent.'

The flowers were rather awful: gladioli and enormous white daisies that looked artificial, and tightly budded roses fanned out behind windows of cellophane. And a couple of wreaths of shiny, hard-looking leaves. These offerings had ridden in the hearse and were stacked now outside the church door. Helen hoped they would not be brought back to the house: she was vague about what the etiquette was here. She longed to be rid of the flowers, of the appalling hours that loomed in which she must dispense hospitality and talk to people, of the whole disagreeable day. She simply wanted to get on with life, which would now be different. She wanted, quite dispassionately, to see what this difference would be. She was also extremely tired. Her mother had died indignantly and demandingly. Neither she nor Edward had had much sleep for quite a while.

And out now into the churchyard, trailing behind the coffin. The hole; the pile of fresh-dug earth. Oh God, thought Helen, this is too awful. Why isn't she being cremated? She is not being cremated because she specified that it should be like this. All in black and white, it appears. Burial in the churchyard of St Peter's, Long Sydenham, in a plot in the far corner near the big sycamore that she laid claim to several years ago, apparently—after, it emerges, a row with the rector that none of us knew a thing about. Now I know why he's been giving us funny looks for so long. So mother envisaged us all here, gathered round staring down in this ghastly way, looking at anything rather than each other, wishing they'd get on and get it over. You could have spared us that, mother.

Earth to earth, ashes to ashes, dust to dust. The words, in fact, are beautiful—

the rhythms, the resonance. The meaning is another matter, for us unbelievers. Mercifully. Eternal life is an appalling idea, especially in mother's case.

And that, at last, was that. They could start to turn away, look at each other, they could leave her there under the sycamore and go. And now, damn and blast it, Helen feels tears prick her eyes, surge up, begin to trickle—and she looks at Edward and sees that he is the same. They both scowl and furtively dab. We can't leave her here, thinks Helen, we can't just put her in there and leave her. Mother.

But they can. And do. She is dead. Helen thinks, almost for the first time, mother has died. She is not here any more. Incredulous, she searches the group around the grave: Edward, Louise, Tim, Suzanne and Phil. No mother, any more.

Evelyn Waugh
1903–1966

From *The Loved One*

DENNIS passed through and opening the door marked 'Inquiries' found himself in a raftered banqueting-hall. 'The Hindu Love-song' was here also, gently discoursed from the dark-oak panelling. A young lady rose from a group of her fellows to welcome him, one of that new race of exquisite, amiable, efficient young ladies whom he had met everywhere in the United States. She wore a white smock and over her sharply supported left breast was embroidered the words, *Mortuary Hostess*.

'Can I help you in any way?'

'I came to arrange about a funeral.'

'Is it for yourself?'

'Certainly not. Do I look so moribund?'

'Pardon me?'

'Do I look as if I were about to die?'

'Why, no. Only many of our friends like to make Before Need Arrangements. Will you come this way?'

She led him through the hall into a soft passage. The *décor* here was Georgian. The 'Hindu Love-song' came to its end and was succeeded by the voice of a nightingale. In a little chintzy parlour he and his hostess sat down to make their arrangements.

'I must first record the Essential Data.'

He told her his name and Sir Francis's.

'Now, Mr Barlow, what had you in mind? Embalmment of course, and after that incineration or not, according to taste. Our crematory is on scientific principles, the heat is so intense that all inessentials are volatilized. Some people did not like the thought that ashes of the casket and clothing were mixed with the Loved One's. Normal disposal is by inhumement, entombment, inurnment, or immurement, but many people just lately prefer insarcophagusment. That is *very* individual. The casket is placed inside a sealed sarcophagus, marble or bronze, and rests permanently above ground in a niche in the mausoleum, with or without a personal stained-glass window above. That, of course, is for those with whom price is not a primary consideration.'

Dennis made no hasty choice. He studied all that was for sale; even the simplest of these coffins, he humbly recognized, outshone the most gorgeous product of the Happier Hunting Ground and when he approached the 2,000-dollar level—and these were not the costliest—he felt himself in the Egypt of the Pharaohs. At length he decided on a massive chest of walnut with bronze enrichments and an interior of quilted satin. Its lid, as recommended, was in two parts.

'You are sure that they will be able to make him presentable?'

'We had a Loved One last month who was found drowned. He had been in the ocean a month and they only identified him by his wrist-watch. They fixed that stiff,' said the hostess disconcertingly lapsing from the high diction she had hitherto employed, 'so he looked like it was his wedding day. The boys up there surely know their job. Why, if he'd sat on an atom bomb, they'd make him presentable.'

'That's very comforting.'

'I'll say it is.' And then slipping on her professional manner again as though it were a pair of glasses, she resumed. 'How will the Loved One be attired? We have our own tailoring section. Sometimes after a very long illness there are not suitable clothes available and sometimes the Waiting Ones think it a waste of a good suit. You see, we can fit a Loved One out very reasonably as a casket-suit does not have to be designed for hard wear and in cases where only the upper part is exposed for leave-taking there is no need for more than jacket and vest. Something dark is best to set off the flowers.'

Dennis was entirely fascinated. At length he said: 'Sir Francis was not much of a dandy. I doubt of his having anything quite suitable for casket wear. But in Europe, I think, we usually employ a shroud.'

'Oh, we have shrouds too. I'll show you some.'

The hostess led him to a set of sliding shelves like a sacristy chest where vestments are stored, and drawing one out revealed a garment such as Dennis had never seen before. Observing his interest she held it up for his closer inspection. It was in appearance like a suit of clothes, buttoned in front but open down the back; the sleeves hung loose, open at the seam; half an inch of linen appeared at the cuff and the V of the waistcoat was similarly filled; a knotted bowtie emerged from the opening of a collar which also lay as though slit from behind. It was the apotheosis of the 'dickey'.

'A speciality of our own,' she said, 'though it is now widely imitated. The idea came from the quick-change artists of vaudeville. It enables one to dress the Loved One without disturbing the pose.'

'Most remarkable. I believe that is just the article we require.'

'With or without trousers?'

'What precisely is the advantage of trousers?'

'For Slumber Room wear. It depends whether you wish the leave-taking to be on the chaise-longue or in the casket.'

'Perhaps I had better see the Slumber Room before deciding.'

'You're welcome.'

She led him out to the hall and up a staircase. The nightingale had now given place to the organ and strains of Handel followed them to the Slumber Floor. Here she asked a colleague, 'Which room have we free?'

'Only Daffodil.'

'This way, Mr Barlow.'

They passed many closed doors of pickled oak until at length she opened one and stood aside for him to enter. He found a little room, brightly furnished and papered. It might have been part of a luxurious modern country club in all its features save one. Bowls of flowers stood disposed about a chintz sofa and on the sofa lay what seemed to be the wax effigy of an elderly woman dressed as though for an evening party. Her white gloved hands held a bouquet and on her nose glittered a pair of rimless pince-nez.

'Oh,' said the guide, 'how foolish of me. We've come into Primrose by mistake. This,' she added superfluously, 'is occupied.'

'Yes.'

'The leave-taking is not till the afternoon but we had better go before one of the cosmeticians finds us. They like to make a few final adjustments before Waiting Ones are admitted. Still, it gives you an idea of the chaise-longue arrangement. We usually recommend the casket half-exposure for gentlemen because the legs never look so well.'

She led him out.

'Will there be many for the leave-taking?'

'Yes, I rather think so, a great many.'

'Then you had better have a suite with an ante-room. The Orchid Room is the best. Shall I make a reservation for that?'

'Yes, do.'

'And the half-exposure in the casket, not the chaise-longue?'

'Not the chaise-longue.'

She led him back towards the reception room.

'It may seem a little strange to you, Mr Barlow, coming on a Loved One unexpectedly in that way.'

'I confess it did a little.'

'You will find it quite different on the day. The leave-taking is a very, very great source of consolation. Often the Waiting Ones last saw their Loved One on a bed of pain surrounded by all the gruesome concomitants of the sick room or the hospital. Here they see them as they knew them in buoyant life, transfigured with peace and happiness. At the funeral they have time only for a last look as they file past. Here in the Slumber Room they can stand as long as they like photographing a last beautiful memory on the mind.'

She spoke, he observed, partly by the book, in the words of the Dreamer, partly in her own brisk language. They were back in the reception room now and she spoke briskly. 'Well, I guess I've got all I want out of you, Mr Barlow, except your signature to the order and a deposit.'

Dennis had come prepared for this. It was part of the Happier Hunting Ground procedure. He paid her 500 dollars and took her receipt.

'Now one of our cosmeticians is waiting to see you and get *her* Essential Data, but before we part may I interest you in our Before Need Provision Arrangements?'

'Everything about Whispering Glades interests me profoundly, but that aspect, perhaps, less than others.'

W. D. Smith
(dates unknown)
E. N. Catlin
(dates unknown)

Ring the Bell Softly

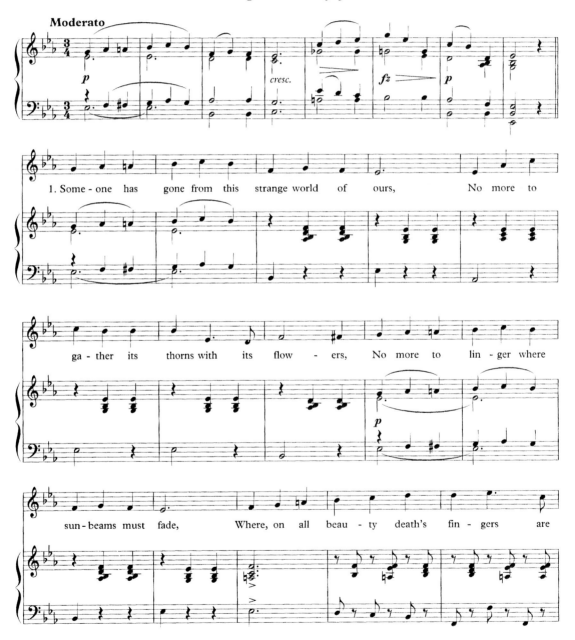

1. Some - one has gone from this strange world of ours, No more to ga - ther its thorns with its flow - ers, No more to lin - ger where sun - beams must fade, Where, on all beau - ty death's fin - gers are

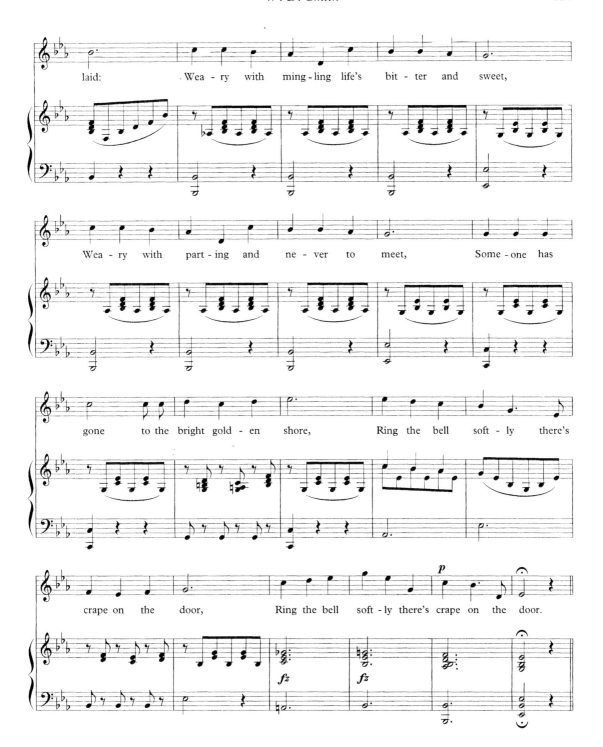

laid: Wea - ry with ming - ling life's bit - ter and sweet,

Wea - ry with part - ing and ne - ver to meet,   Some - one has

gone   to the bright gold - en   shore,   Ring the bell soft - ly there's

crape on the   door,   Ring the bell soft - ly there's crape on the door.

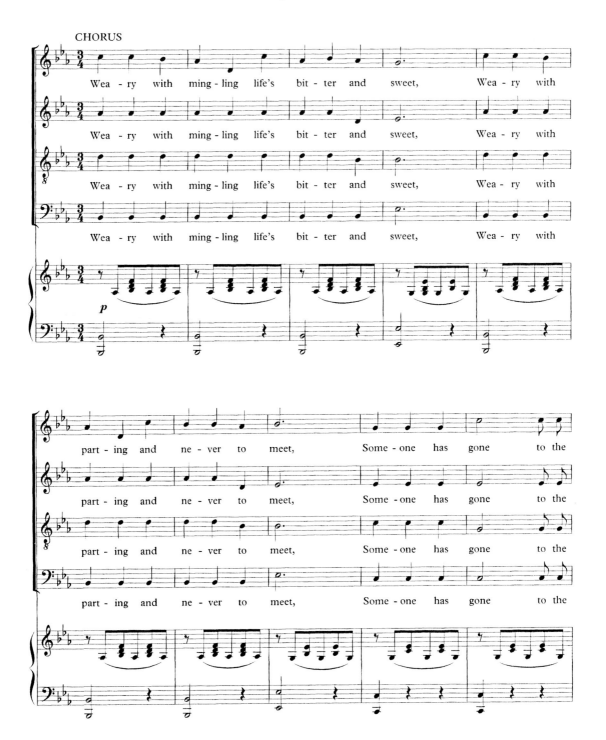

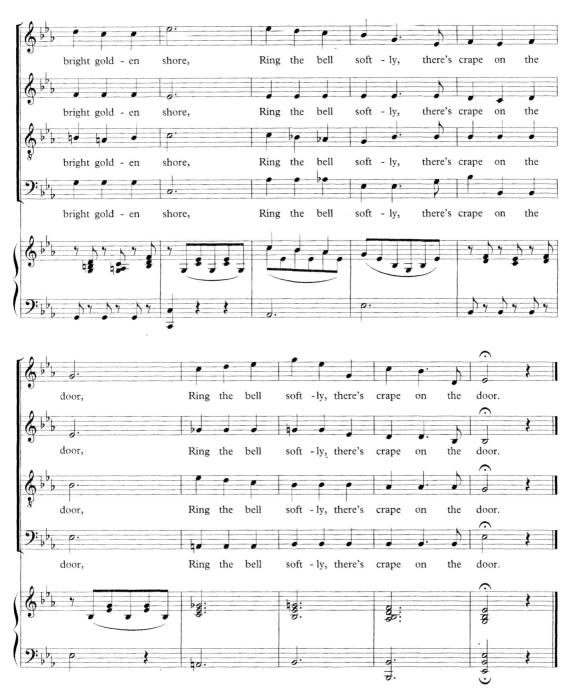

[*Editor's Note:* This song illustrates the enjoyment the Victorians obtained from mourning. The melody is restrained, until the composer breaks out with an exuberant high G in the third last bar of the chorus.]

C. S. Lewis
1898–1963

A Grief Observed

No one ever told me that grief felt so like fear. I am not afraid, but the sensation is like being afraid. The same fluttering in the stomach, the same restlessness, the yawning. I keep on swallowing.

At other times it feels like being mildly drunk, or concussed. There is a sort of invisible blanket between the world and me. I find it hard to take in what anyone says. Or perhaps, hard to want to take it in. It is so uninteresting. Yet I want the others to be about me. I dread the moments when the house is empty. If only they would talk to one another and not to me.

There are moments, most unexpectedly, when something inside me tries to assure me that I don't really mind so much, not so very much, after all. Love is not the whole of a man's life. I was happy before I ever met H. I've plenty of what are called 'resources'. People get over these things. Come, I shan't do so badly. One is ashamed to listen to this voice but it seems for a little to be making out a good case. Then comes a sudden jab of red-hot memory and all this 'commonsense' vanishes like an ant in the mouth of a furnace.

On the rebound one passes into tears and pathos. Maudlin tears. I almost prefer the moments of agony. These are at least clean and honest. But the bath of self-pity, the wallow, the loathsome sticky-sweet pleasure of indulging it—that disgusts me. And even while I'm doing it I know it leads me to misrepresent H. herself. Give that mood its head and in a few minutes I shall have substituted for the real woman a mere doll to be blubbered over. Thank God the memory of her is still too strong (will it always be too strong?) to let me get away with it.

For H. wasn't like that at all. Her mind was lithe and quick and muscular as a leopard. Passion, tenderness, and pain were all equally unable to disarm it. It scented the first whiff of cant or slush; then sprang, and knocked you over before you knew what was happening. How many bubbles of mine she pricked! I soon learned not to talk rot to her unless I did it for the sheer pleasure—and there's another red-hot jab—of being exposed and laughed at. I was never less silly than as H's lover.

And no one ever told me about the laziness of grief. Except at my job—where the machine seems to run on much as usual—I loathe the slightest effort. Not only writing but even reading a letter is too much. Even shaving. What does it matter now whether my cheek is rough or smooth? They say an unhappy man wants distractions—something to take him out of himsclf. Only as a dog-tired man wants an extra blanket on a cold night; he'd rather lie there shivering than get up and find one. It's easy to see why the lonely become untidy; finally, dirty and disgusting.

Meanwhile, where is God? This is one of the most disquieting symptoms. When you are happy, so happy that you have no sense of needing Him, so happy that you are tempted to feel His claims upon you as an interruption, if you remember yourself and turn to Him with gratitude and praise, you will be—or so it feels—welcomed with open arms. But go to Him when your need is desperate, when all other help is vain, and what do you find? A door slammed in your face, and a sound of bolting and double bolting on the inside. After that, silence. You may as well turn away. The longer you wait, the more emphatic the silence will become. There are no lights in the windows. It might be an empty house. Was it ever inhabited? It seemed so once. And that seeming was as strong as this. What can this mean? Why is He so present a commander in our time of prosperity and so very absent a help in time of trouble?

I tried to put some of these thoughts to C. this afternoon. He reminded me that the same thing seems to have happened to Christ: 'Why hast thou forsaken me?' I know. Does that make it easier to understand?

Not that I am (I think) in much danger of ceasing to believe in God. The real danger is of coming to believe such dreadful things about Him. The conclusion I dread is not 'So there's no God after all,' but 'So this is what God's really like. Deceive yourself no longer.'

Our elders submitted and said 'Thy will be done.' How often had bitter resentment been stifled through sheer terror and an act of love—yes, in every sense, an act—put on to hide the operation?

Of course it's easy enough to say that God seems absent at our greatest need because He *is* absent—non-existent. But then why does He seem so present when, to put it quite frankly, we don't ask for Him?

One thing, however, marriage has done for me. I can never again believe that religion is manufactured out of our unconscious, starved desires and is a substitute for sex. For those few years H. and I feasted on love; every mode of it—solemn and merry, romantic and realistic, sometimes as dramatic as a thunderstorm, sometimes as comfortable and unemphatic as putting on your soft slippers. No cranny of heart or body remained unsatisfied. If God were a substitute for love we ought to have lost all interest in Him. Who'd bother about substitutes when he has the thing itself? But that isn't what happens. We both knew we wanted something besides one another—quite a different kind of something, a quite different kind of want. You might as well say that when lovers have one another they will never want to read, or eat—or breathe.

After the death of a friend, years ago, I had for some time a most vivid feeling of certainty about his continued life; even his enhanced life. I have begged to be given even one hundredth part of the same assurance about H. There is no answer. Only the locked door, the iron curtain, the vacuum, absolute zero. 'Them as asks don't get.' I was a fool to ask. For now, even if that assurance came I should distrust it. I should think it a self-hypnosis induced by my own prayers.

At any rate I must keep clear of the spiritualists. I promised H. I would. She knew something of those circles.

Keeping promises to the dead, or to anyone else, is very well. But I begin to see that 'respect for the wishes of the dead' is a trap. Yesterday I stopped myself only in time from saying about some trifle 'H. wouldn't have liked that.' This is unfair to the others. I should soon be using 'what H. would have liked' as an instrument of domestic tyranny; with her supposed likings becoming a thinner and thinner disguise for my own.

I cannot talk to the children about her. The moment I try, there appears on their faces neither grief, nor love, nor fear, nor pity, but the most fatal of all non-conductors, embarrassment. They look as if I were committing an indecency. They are longing for me to stop. I felt just the same after my own mother's death when my father mentioned her. I can't blame them. It's the way boys are.

I sometimes think that shame, mere awkward, senseless shame, does as much towards preventing good acts and straightforward happiness as any of our vices can do. And not only in boyhood.

Or are the boys right? What would H. herself think of this terrible little notebook to which I come back and back? Are these jottings morbid? I once read the sentence 'I lay awake all night with toothache, thinking about toothache and about lying awake.' That's true to life. Part of every misery is, so to speak, the misery's shadow or reflection: the fact that you don't merely suffer but have to keep on thinking about the fact that you suffer. I not only live each endless day in grief, but live each day thinking about living each day in grief. Do these notes merely aggravate that side of it? Merely confirm the monotonous, tread-mill march of the mind round one subject? But what am I to do? I must have some drug, and reading isn't a strong enough drug now. By writing it all down (all?—no: one thought in a hundred) I believe I get a little outside it. That's how I'd defend it to H. But ten to one she'd see a hole in the defence.

Wendy Cope
1945–

An Unusual Cat-Poem

My cat is dead
But I have decided not to make a big tragedy out of it.

✥7✥

Research

*U*NCERTAINTY *of diagnosis, treatment, and prognosis are inevitable in medicine, and the only way ahead is through research. There have been notable advances, such as William Harvey's discovery of the circulation of the blood, but many less successful investigations. One of these is amusingly described by Richard Asher. Individual doctors and all others involved in health care—I have chosen a doctor and a pharmacist— must keep their own ideas up to date, and the passages selected make it clear that this is not always easy. Perhaps it would be easier to keep up to date if professional journals were written in a more lively manner, as Richard Asher suggests.*

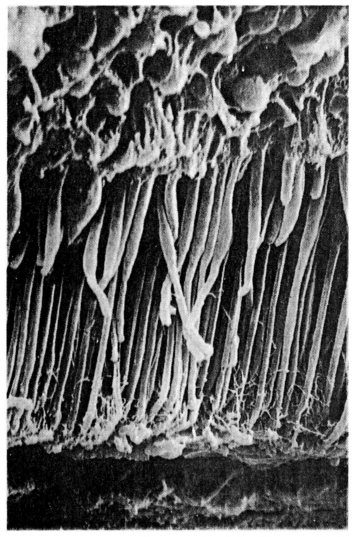

Scanning Electron Micrograph of the Human Retina

In this scanning electron micrograph of the human retina numerous rods and a solitary cone can be seen. Rods are concentrated in the peripheral area of the retina, and they function best in dim lighting conditions and register movement. Cones are concentrated mainly in the central area and are responsible for colour vision. There are three types of cone, one for each of the primary colours (red, blue, and yellow). Colour perception results from a synthesis of these primary colour messages in much the same way as the artist mixes colours on the palette. It is also interesting to consider how far an image of this sort, created for scientific purposes, can at the same time be considered a work of art.

Uncertainty

Hippocrates
c.460–357 BC

From *Aphorisms*

LIFE is short, science is long; opportunity is elusive, experience is dangerous, judgement is difficult. It is not enough for the physician to do what is necessary, but the patient and the attendants must do their part as well, and circumstances must be favourable.

(*Translated from the Greek by J. Chadwick and W. N. Mann*)

Ben Jonson
1572–1637

From *An Anatomy of the World*

THOU art too narrow, wretch, to comprehend
Even thyself, yea though thou wouldst but bend
To know thy body. Have not all souls thought
For many ages, that our bodies wrought
Of air, and fire, and other elements?
And now they think of new ingredients;
And one soul thinks one, and another way
Another thinks, and 'tis an even lay.
Know'st thou but how the stone doth enter in
The bladder's cave, and never break the skin?

Know'st thou how blood, which to the heart doth flow,
Doth from one ventricle to th' other go?
And for the putrid stuff which thou dost spit,
Know'st thou how thy lungs have attracted it?
There are no passages, so that there is
—For aught thou know'st—piercing of substances.
And of those many opinions which men raise
Of nails and hairs, dost thou know which to praise?
What hope have we to know ourselves, when we
Know not the least things which for our use be?

Hilaire Belloc
1870–1953

The Microbe

THE microbe is so very small
You cannot make him out at all,
But many sanguine people hope
To see him through a microscope.
His jointed tongue that lies beneath
A hundred curious rows of teeth;
His seven tufted tails with lots
Of lovely pink and purple spots,
On each of which a pattern stands,
Composed of forty separate bands;
His eyebrows of a tender green;
All these have never yet been seen—
But Scientists, who ought to know,
Assure us that they must be so . . .
Oh! let us never, never doubt
What nobody is sure about!

Philip Larkin
1922–1985

Ignorance

STRANGE to know nothing, never to be sure
Of what is true or right or real,
But forced to qualify *or so I feel*,
Or *Well, it does seem so*:
Someone must know

Strange to be ignorant of the way things work:
Their skill at finding what they need,
Their sense of shape, and punctual spread of seed,
And willingness to change;
Yes, it is strange,

Even to wear such knowledge—for our flesh
Surrounds us with its own decisions—
And yet spend all our life on imprecisions,
That when we start to die
Have no idea why.

The Pursuit of Knowledge

John Aubrey
1625–1697

From *Brief Lives*

[*The Circulation of the Blood*]

WILLIAM HARVEY [1578–1659]; Dr of Physique and Chirurgery, Inventor of the Circulation of the Bloud, was borne at the house which is now the Posthouse, a faire stone-built-house, which he gave to Caius College in Cambridge, with some lands there. His brother Eliab would have given any money or exchange for it, because 'twas his father's, and they all borne there; but the Doctor (truly) thought his memory would better be preserved this way, for his brother has left noble seates, and about 3,000 pounds per annum at least.

William Harvey was always very contemplative, and the first that I heare of that was curious in Anatomie in England. I remember I have heard him say he wrote a booke *De Insectis*, which he had been many yeares about, and had made dissections of Frogges, Toades, and a number of other Animals, and had made curious Observations on them, which papers, together with his goods, in his Lodgings at Whitehall, were plundered at the beginning of the Rebellion, he being for the King, and with him at Oxon; but he often sayd, That of all the losses he sustained, no griefe was so crucifying to him as the losse of these papers, which for love or money he could never retrive or obtaine.

When Charles I by reason of the Tumults left London, he attended him, and was at the fight of Edge-hill with him; and during the fight, the Prince and Duke of Yorke were committed to his care. He told me that he withdrew with them under a hedge, and tooke out of his pockett a booke and read; but he had not read very long before a Bullet of a great Gun grazed on the ground neare him, which made him remove his station.

He told me that Sir Adrian Scrope was dangerously wounded there, and left for dead amongst the dead men, stript; which happened to be the saving of his Life. It was cold, cleer weather, and a frost that night; which staunched his bleeding, and about midnight, or some houres after his hurte, he awaked, and was faine to drawe a dead body upon him for warmeth-sake.

I first sawe him at Oxford, 1642, after Edgehill fight, but was then too young to be acquainted with so great a Doctor. I remember he came severall times to Trinity College to George Bathurst, B.D., who had a Hen to hatch Egges in his chamber, which they dayly opened to discerne the progres and way of Generation. I had not the honour to be acquainted with him till 1651, being my she cosen Montague's physitian and friend. I was at that time bound for Italy (but to my great griefe disswaded by my mother's importunity). He was very communicative, and willing to instruct any that were modest and respectfull to him. And in order to my Journey, gave me, i.e. dictated to me, what to see, what company to keepe, what Bookes to read, how to manage my Studies: in short, he bid me goe to the Fountain head, and read Aristotle, Cicero, Avicenna, and did call the Neoteriques shitt-breeches.

He wrote a very bad hand, which (with use) I could pretty well read. He understood Greek and Latin pretty well, but was no Critique, and he wrote very bad Latin. The *Circuitis Sanguinis* [Circulation of the Blood] was, as I take it, donne into Latin by Sir George Ent.

At Oxford, he grew acquainted with Dr Charles Scarborough, then a young Physitian (since by King Charles II Knighted) in whose conversation he much delighted; and whereas before, he marched up and downe with the Army, he tooke him to him and made him ly in his Chamber, and said to him, Prithee leave off thy gunning, and stay here; I will bring thee into practice.

His Majestie King Charles I gave him the Wardenship of Merton Colledge in Oxford, as a reward for his service, but the Times suffered him not to recieve or injoy any benefitt by it.

After Oxford was surrendred, which was 24 July 1646, he came to London, and lived with his brother Eliab a rich Merchant in London, who bought, about 1654, Cockaine-house, now (1680) the Excise-office, a noble house, where the Doctor was wont to contemplate on the Leads of the House, and had his severall stations, in regard of the sun, or wind.

He did delight to be in the darke, and told me he could then best contemplate. He had a house heretofore at Combe, in Surrey, a good aire and prospect, where he had Caves made in the Earth, in which in Summer time he delighted to meditate.

Ah! my old friend Dr Harvey—I knew him right well. He made me sitt by him 2 or 3 hours together in his meditating apartment discoursing. Why, had he been stiffe, starcht, and retired, as other formall Doctors are, he had knowne no more than they. From the meanest person, in some way, or other, the learnedst man may learn something. Pride has been one of the greatest stoppers of the Advancement of Learning.

He was far from Bigotry.

He was wont to say that man was but a great, mischievous Baboon.

He had been physitian to the Lord Chancellour Bacon, whom he esteemed much for his witt and style, but would not allow him to be a great Philosopher. Said he to me, *He writes Philosophy like a Lord Chancellor*, speaking in derision; *I have cured him.*

When Doctor Harvey (one of the Physitians College in London) being a Young Man, went to Travel towards Padoa: he went to Dover (with several others) and shewed his Pass, as the rest did, to the Governor there. The Governor told him, that he must not go, but he must keep him Prisoner. The Doctor desired to know for what reason? how he has transgrest. Well, it was his Will to have it so. The Pacquet Boat Hoised Sail in the Evening (which was very clear) and the Doctor's Companions in it. There ensued a terrible Storme, and the Pacquet Boat and all the Passengers were Drown'd: The next day the sad News was brought to Dover. The Doctor was unknown to the Governor, both by Name and Face; but the Night before the Governor had a perfect Vision in a Dream of Doctor Harvey, who came to pass over to Calais; and that he had a Warning to stop him. This the Governor told to the Doctor the next day. The Doctor was a pious good Man, and has several time directed this Story to some of my Acquaintance.

Dr Harvey told me, and any one if he examines himself will find it to be true, that a man could not fancy—truthfully—that he is imperfect in any part that he has, *verbi gratia*, Teeth, Eie, Tongue, Spina dorsi, etc. Natura tends to perfection, and in matters of Generation we ought to consult more with our sense and instinct, then our reason, and prudence, fashion of the country, and Interest. We see what contemptible products are of the prudent politiques; weake, fooles, and ricketty children, scandalls to nature and their country. The Heralds are fooles: *tota errant via* [they are on completely the wrong track]. A blessing goes with a marriage for love upon a strong impulse.

He that marries a widdowe makes himself Cuckold. *Exempli gratia*, if a good Bitch is first warded with a Curre, let her ever after be warded with a dog of a good straine and yet she will bring curres as at first, her wombe being first infected with a Curre. So, the children will be like the first Husband (like raysing up children to your brother). So, the Adulterer, though a crime in Law, the children are like the husband.

He would say that we Europeans knew not how to order or governe our Woemen, and that the Turks were the only people used them wisely.

I remember he kept a pretty young wench to wayte on him, which I guesse he made use of for warmeth-sake as King David did, and tooke care of her in his Will, as also of his man servant.

He was very Cholerique; and in his young days wore a dagger (as the fashion then was) but this Dr would be to apt to draw-out his dagger upon every slight occasion.

I have heard him say, that after his Booke of the *Circulation of the Blood* came out, that he fell mightily in his Practize, and that 'twas beleeved by the vulgar that he was crack-brained; and all the Physitians were against his Opinion, and envyed [*grudged against*] him; many wrote against him. With much adoe at last, in about 20 or 30 yeares time, it was recieved in all the Universities in the world; and Mr Hobbes sayes in his book *De Corpore* [Of the Body], *he is the only man, perhaps, that ever lived to see his owne Doctrine established in his life-time.*

He was Physitian, and a great Favorite of the Lord High Marshall of England, Thomas Howard Earle of Arundel and Surrey, with whom he travelled as his Physitian in his Ambassade to the Emperor at Vienna. In his Voyage, he would still be making of excursions into the Woods, makeing Observations of strange Trees, and plants, earths, etc., naturalls, and sometimes like to be lost, so that my Lord Ambassador would be really angry with him, for there was not only danger of Thieves, but also of wild beasts.

He was much and often troubled with the Gowte, and his way of Cure was thus; he would then sitt with his Legges bare, if it were a Frost, on the leads of Cockaine-house, putt them into a payle of water, till he was almost dead with cold, and betake himselfe to his Stove, and so 'twas gone.

He was hott-headed, and his thoughts working would many times keepe him from sleepinge; he told me that then his way was to rise out of his Bed and walke about his Chamber in his Shirt till he was pretty coole, i.e. till he began to have a horror, and then returne to bed, and sleepe very comfortably.

He was not tall; but of the lowest stature, round faced, olivaster complexion; little Eie, round, very black, full of spirit; his haire was black as a Raven, but quite white 20 yeares before he dyed.

I remember he was wont to drinke Coffee; which he and his brother Eliab did, before Coffee-houses were in fashion in London.

His practise was not very great towards his later end; he declined it, unlesse to a speciall friend, e.g. my Lady Howland, who had a cancer in her Breast, which he did cutt-off and seared, but at last she dyed of it. He rode on horseback with a

Footcloath [ornamental saddle-cloth] to visitt his Patients, his man following on foote, as the fashion then was, which was very decent, now quite discontinued. (The Judges rode also with their Foote-cloathes to Westminster-hall, which ended at the death of Sir Robert Hyde, Lord Chief Justice. Anthony Earl of Shafton, would have revived, but severall of the judges being old and ill horsemen would not agree to it.)

All his Profession would allow him to be an excellent Anatomist, but I never heard of any that admired his Therapeutique way. I knew severall practisers in London that would not have given 3d. for one of his Bills; and that a man could hardly tell by one of his Bills what he did aime at. (He did not care for Chymistrey, and was wont to speake against them with an undervalue.)

He had, towards his latter end, a preparation of Opium and I know not what, which he kept in his study to take, if occasion should serve, to putt him out of his paine, and which Sir Charles Scarborough promised to give him; this I beleeve to be true; but doe not at all beleeve that he really did give it him.

Not but that, had he laboured under great Paines, he had been readie enough to have donne it; I doe not deny that it was not according to his Principles upon certain occasions. But the manner of his dyeing was really, and *bonâ fide*, thus, viz. the morning of his death about 10 a clock, he went to speake, and found he had the dead palsey in his Tongue; then he sawe what was to become of him, he knew there was then no hopes of his recovery, so presently sends for his brother and young nephewes to come-up to him, to whome he gives one his Watch ('twas a minute watch with which he made his experiments), to another another thing, etc., as remembrances of him; made a signe to Sambroke, his Apothecary, to lett him blood in the Tongue, which did little or no good; and so ended his dayes. The Palsey did give him an easy Passe-port.

For 20 yeares before he dyed he tooke no manner of care about his worldly concernes, but his brother Eliab, who was a very wise and prudent menager, ordered all not only faithfully, but better then he could have donne himselfe. He dyed worth 20,000 pounds, which he left to his brother Eliab. In his Will he left his old friend Mr Thomas Hobbes 10 pounds as a token of his Love.

He lies buried in a Vault at Hempsted in Essex, which his brother Eliab Harvey built; he is lapt in lead, and on his brest in great letters:

DR WILLIAM HARVEY

I was at his Funerall, and helpt to carry him into the Vault.

Richard Asher
1912–1969
Is Baldness Psychological?

A PSYCHOLOGICAL explanation for baldness is not a surprising thing because it is now the fashion for psychiatrists to put forward mental causes for those illnesses where physical mechanisms have not yet been found—for instance, peptic ulcer, rheumatism and others. Szasz and Robertson,[*] a psychoanalyst and psychiatrist, watching their patients' expressions decided that bald men looked more tense than non-bald men; from this observation they worked out 'a new integrated theory of baldness.'

Briefly, they account for baldness thus: a man has a hidden anxiety and a defensive attitude to life This gives him 'a rigid expression, often noticeable as a fixed smile or a toothy smile'. Now, as there is a close association between face and scalp movements (both in nerve supply and development), the chronic tonicity of the facial muscles is reflected in chronic scalp tension, which leads to blood-vessel-pinching effects from shearing stresses on the subcutaneous tissues of the scalp and consequently to loss of hair. In other words, the man who persistently 'puts a brave face on it' is at the same time starving his hair of its blood supply. Wilhelmina Stitch wrote: 'It is easy enough to be pleasant when life goes by like a song, but the man worth while is the man who will smile when everything goes dead wrong.' Perhaps these words, so often hung in poker work upon a living room wall, may have unwittingly caused a good many hairs to be shed, for the 'smile when everything goes dead wrong' is just that rigid smile which Szasz and Robertson accuse of causing that scalp distortion which leads to baldness; indeed, a famous marching song of the Great War may have produced many bald soldiers, and if we had our songs first vetted by psychiatrists (as perhaps we should) we might be bidden: 'Pack up your troubles in the old kit bag and relax, relax, relax.' They quote Wilhelm Reich,[†] who considers such smiles 'a somatic character armour'. 'The psychological defences of a neurotic personality which serve as a protection from feelings of insecurity and anxiety.' They also point out that tightening of the scalp may occur with a defensive attitude to life just as animals that fight with their teeth draw back their ears when savage to prevent them from being torn by their antagonists (Darwin)[‡] and tighten their scalps to prevent their

---

[*] T. S. Szasz and A. M. Robertson. *Arch. Derm. Syph. Chicago*, 61 (1950), 34–48.

[†] W. Reich, *Character Analysis*, 2nd edn. (New York: Orgone Institute Press, 1945).

[‡] C. Darwin, *The Expressions of the Emotions in Man and Animals* (New York: Appleton and Co, 1898).

opponents from seizing a loose piece of skin. In other words, the bald individual may be one who has tightened his scalp lest fate should take a nip at it, and ordinary alopecia may represent the result of a chronic and concealed snarl at life.

This is an intriguing idea and ingeniously worked out, but it is wise to remember Clifford Allbutt's words, 'the use of hypotheses lies not in the display of ingenuity, but in the labour of verification', and much more convincing evidence would have to be forthcoming for the theory to become widely accepted. At the start the original observation that bald men wore fixed expressions might be tested more scientifically by confronting the psychiatrists with a large number of photographs of faces which had their scalps concealed and seeing if they could pick out the bald heads by studying their expressions. Some explanation would also have to be found for the fact that people with one sided facial tics are not observed to have unilateral baldness, although the shearing stresses on the scalp from repeated grimacing must be much greater than those due to a fixed tense expression. The professional strong man too—for ever rippling his pectoral muscles at the circus— might be expected to epilate his sternal region by a similar mechanism, but the hairy chests of such persons are in fact proverbial.

Only two things about ordinary baldness seem to be agreed upon by all observers. First, that it is almost unknown in women, and secondly, that it is often hereditary. Szasz and Robertson manage to fit these observations neatly into their scheme. They attribute women's immunity to baldness to the thicker fat padding in their scalps, which protects the blood vessels against shearing stress (it has been shown that testosterone accounts for the thinner fatty layer in men, and J. B. Hamilton* claimed to produce baldness in eunuchs by giving testosterone). They account for the genetic factors in baldness by saying they predispose to certain skull shapes which favour the development of greater tension of the scalp, or possibly by 'determining affinities for more archaic kinds of muscular expression'. The second idea is the more intriguing because it suggests that if our inward tension gets the better of us we might revert to an archaic expression with teeth bared and ears drawn back and so begin to get thin on top. Looking at distinguished doctors at a medical meeting it is hard to take this view when we note those placid professional faces which are so often topped by polished domes, but perhaps they may have borne more archaic expressions in the past. Certainly the schoolboy who bids his companion to restrain his temper says 'keep your hair on', and if we are to believe Szasz and Robertson this boyish phrase is no meaningless expression but a medical warning based on psychiatric theory.

* J. B. Hamilton, *Am. J. Anat.* 71 (1942), 451–80.

Szasz and Robertson attempted to confirm their theory by electromyographic studies of bald and non-bald men. They measured the electrical activity of the occipitalis, expecting the bald subjects to show a continuous action of this muscle, but the bald men were able to relax their scalps as easily as their better covered colleagues. No significant difference in the electromyograms of the two groups was found, but the record voltage (over 1 volt) was registered by a non-bald man wiggling his ears. Despite the negative results of this experiment the authors feel that further research should be done to verify their theory. They suggest submitting the bald subject to more searching procedures, but one cannot help feeling that if a bald man knew that there was a plan to cut the nerves to his scalp, inject radioactive substances into the blood vessels of his hair, fix electrodes to his head throughout the night, and finally to psychoanalyse him, he might develop such a degree of inward tension and such a distortion of the normal facial expression as to interfere materially with the proper scientific conduct of the experiment. Perhaps the average bald man would prefer to buy himself a hat.

(From *Clinical Excerpts*, April–June 1951)

Brian Sheldon
1944–
A Pharmaceutical Nightmare

ONE day a dispensary student had been left to mind the store and was confronted unexpectedly by a customer asking for a convenient remedy for aching feet. Anxious to approach the problem systematically rather than just handing over any old type of ointment, the student retired to the back room and looked up 'Feet (sore)' in the still pristine volumes of his *Theory and Practice for Pharmacy Students*. Here he discovered that the condition could seemingly be caused (although the authors are cautious in their use of that word), by anything from tightly fitting shoes to Intermittent Claudication. Disconcertingly, his book offered little guidance as to 'most likely explanations'. New suggestions about how to approach such problems had been slotted in alongside the old (some of these undoubtedly dating back to the alchemists) and no remedy had ever really gone out of date, or could be said to have been 'replaced' with something more effective. More worryingly, each of the aetiological accounts presented seemed logically to rule out all the others, but then this seemed to worry none of the contributors— least of all the editors.

Not understanding how he was expected to make use of such a guide, our student sought the author's preface. Here he was confronted with the view that given the 'uniqueness' of each of the conditions reported on, the ultimate choice had to be left to the individual dispenser: 'it all depends what works for you' ran the relevant paragraph.

Closing the book, and filled with a new enthusiasm, he reflected momentarily on his previous misconception. They were right of course, he should have realized where his appetite for practical prescription was leading him; to theoretical synthesis, comparative evaluation of concepts, cumulative collections of theory, and the like. Mechanistic impositions on the freedom and creativity of the man at the practice interface. Much better to guess—flexibly and intuitively of course. He remembered from his lectures on Non-Directive Pharmacy the dangers attaching to the indiscriminate use of 'narrow empirical products', Jehu's Jelly, Skinner's Salve, and such. No, he must not seek to avoid his professional responsibilities, the choice was his alone. However, on returning to his shelves to look intuitively for likely remedies, he was faced with another setback. From the accompanying literature he discerned that most of the available mixtures had never been tested at all. Those which had were far from spectacular successes he recalled, and had only been kept on the market for the sake of a few addicts. Just then our hovering student's attention was caught by a large volume sitting on the topmost shelf. It was entitled 'Feet and Society'. A quick translation from it revealed that sore feet result from interaction with Pedestrian Transportation Facilities (pavements, as they are sometimes called by the non-technical). Furthermore, structural factors in late capitalist society determine that profit-motivated footwear suppliers are forced increasingly to skimp on their products at the expense of the oppressed consumer.

The student dashed from his dispensary eager to raise the consciousness of his customer with this new knowledge, but alas, she had tired of waiting and hobbled away.

William Carlos Williams
1883–1963

Le Médecin Malgré Lui

OH I suppose I should
wash the walls of my office
polish the rust from
my instruments and keep them
definitely in order
build shelves in the laboratory
empty out the old stains
clean the bottles
and refill them, buy
another lens, put
my journals on edge instead of
letting them lie flat
in heaps—then begin
ten years back and
gradually
read them to date
cataloguing important
articles for ready reference.
I suppose I should
read the new books.
If to this I added
a bill at the tailor's
and at the cleaner's
grew a decent beard
and cultivated a look
of importance—
Who can tell? I might be
a credit to my Lady Happiness
and never think anything
but a white thought!

Writing Up

Richard Asher
1912–1969

Why Are Medical Journals So Dull?

MEDICAL journals are dull; I do not think there is any doubt about that. There are many causes of their dullness; some are curable and some incurable. I do not separate them: this is a short study of the pathology, not a dissertation on the prophylaxis and treatment, of the condition.

WRAPPERS AND COVERS

Their wrappings are drab and difficult to remove, so the journals accumulate on our desks in inconvenient piles and roll on to the floor. There is little incentive to make the effort of opening them. When opened they have a strong tendency to roll themselves up again.

The covers are as drab as the wrappers. There is nothing on the cover to distinguish one copy from another or to titillate the clinical appetite. There is in some journals a table of contents on the outside page, but the titles are so discouraging that they provide very little incentive for reading the journal, especially to a man already weakened by the effort of unwrapping and correctively rerolling the twisted pages. In other journals the table of contents is hidden among the first few pages of advertisements. Advertisers pay more if their wares are inserted half way through the programme, as in commercial television, and so while hopefully scanning the contents one is interrupted by a vasodilator or a purgative. With the *Proceedings of the Royal Society of Medicine* I have quite often missed something because an advertisement made me think I had finished the list of contents.

TITLES

Many of the titles are unattractive. Without going in for sensationalism an author can try to make his title allure as well as inform. A medical journal is an open market where each salesman must cry his goods if he wishes to get an audience at his stall. A poor title dulls the clinical appetite, whereas a good title whets it. I have called this article 'Why are Medical Journals so Dull?' I do not claim this title is specially good, but it is better than 'A Study of the Negativistic Psychomotor Reactions induced by Perusal of Verbalized Clinical Materials'. Titles such as 'A Trial of 4.4-Diethyl-hydro-balderdashic Acid in Acute Coryzal Infections' are far better changed to 'A New Treatment for Colds'.

An important addition to the title should be the author's name, which may attract or repel according to the reputation he enjoys; but medical articles today often appear to be written by committees, and this multiple authorship is highly discouraging to readers. Ten men cannot write an article any more than ten men can drive a car. The interest evoked by an author's name is diluted by listing all his advisers.

WANTING IN COLOUR

So much for the cover. Now for the inside. The paper is often of poor quality, and coloured pictures are almost unknown. I realize it is economically impossible that this should be otherwise, but medical journals contrast so glumly with the glossy productions of the big drug houses or with women's weeklies.

The advertisements in medical journals are essential to add revenue, but they add little else and seem far less exciting than the advertisements in lay weeklies. Prosperous people in brightly coloured dresses sipping expensive drinks in luxurious liners provide us with happy daydreams of holidays we cannot afford. Advertisements in medical journals are quite the reverse: elderly men in shabby pyjamas hurrying along the passage with urinary frequency. They are not attractive; nor are the other afflicted persons pictured there with tension, hypertension, insomnia, and pain. Humorous advertisements in medical advertising are rare; it might be cheering to see a strip cartoon of the doctor whose practice dwindled because of night starvation but rose with dramatic success after Horlicks; or the physician who found his failure to be elected to fellowship was due to his not using Amplex.

In short, there are many factors which dull the prospect of reading a medical journal even before the letterpress is reached: the wrapping, the unwrapping, the titles, the authors, and the advertisements. There are additional psychological deterrents—the feeling of duty: 'I ought to read this for my exams; for my edification; to keep up with my houseman; because my patients will read it in the *Reader's Digest*; or because George will ask me what I think of it. Duty, if one is aware of it, is usually a deterrent, but it is also associated with the idea that a lot of what you don't fancy does you good.

A TEDIOUS DUTY

Now for the letterpress itself. It is inevitable that editors have to accept a certain amount of junk both to fill their papers and to avoid giving offence to eminent medical men. For many doctors the achievement of a published article is a tedious duty to be surmounted as a necessary hurdle in a medical career. You have got to get over it, just as you have to dissect a dogfish for the first MB; you don't like it, but it's got to be done. Though the subject of an article is important, it is not much to do with its dullness. I believe that if a man has something to say which interests him, and he knows how to say it, then he need never be dull. Unfortunately, some people have a desire for publication but nothing more. They have nothing to say, and they do not know how to say it. They want to be seen in the *British Medical Journal* or the *Lancet* because it is respectable to be seen there, like being seen in church. They would stand no chance of publication in lay magazines, but the number of medical magazines is so large that every dull dog has his day. Often there seems to be a spate of articles on the same subject: for example, intervertebral discs were all the rage some years ago, whereas hiatus hernia is much in the news today. Other subjects, especially in the correspondence columns, flower, like cacti, every two or three years: for instance, discussions on herpes zoster and chickenpox, or on the correct use of 'tropic' and 'trophic'.

GOOD PRESENTATION

The dullness of an article depends much on its presentation—that is, the way it is set out, the order in which the facts are put, and the way the diagrams or pictures are arranged. It is astonishing what a difference this makes. For example, here are two ways of setting out one case. A man was crushed by a bombed building, injuring his diaphragm. He consequently developed a right diaphragmatic hernia which resulted in dyspepsia from visceral displacement. Surgical repair of the hernia relieved his symptoms.

That account is factual and accurate, but not especially interesting. Here is the same case as I heard it described by the surgeon at a meeting of a clinical section. He operated on a man who had symptoms of duodenal ulcers, and to his chagrin was unable to deliver the duodenum. At length his exploring hands disappeared into a large hole in the right diaphragm, where he found much intestine. There was no duodenal ulcer. He then reviewed the chest x-ray film and found that the alleged thickened pleura was really hernia and that gas could be (and should have been) recognized in it. As soon as the man came round from the operation a fresh history was taken, and it was found that the pain was nothing like ulcer pain; it had no periodicity (it had been caused by the duodenum being stretched across the lumbar spine). Also, the history of the crush injury was elicited; until then it had not been discovered. The surgeon concluded: 'The moral is that one ought to take a history before the operation rather than after it.'

You will agree that this second version is live: the first was dead. The first was chronological and factual, yet was tidied up so much that there was no interest left: it had the dullness of a sieved diet.

May I mention a recently published case of my own, 'A Woman with the Stiff-Man Syndrome'? Here I wrote the accounts of events not in chronological order but in logical order, starting with my reading an annotation on this syndrome, then my realizing I had seen a case of it ten years previously, then a search for the lady, followed by a review of the notes, and finally a description of her behaviour at a clinical meeting. I thought this would make the article more alive. This device of telling a story by starting in the present and darting to the past and back is far from original, yet to my surprise I received a large number of approving letters and telephone calls praising the way the article was written. I did not know so many people minded about presentation. The amount of comment produced when trouble was taken to make the presentation as interesting as possible suggests that the average contribution may be rather dull in presentation and that a lively contribution shines like a good deed in a naughty world. I am sure many people writing for medical journals would take more trouble if they knew how much difference it made.

To refer to an article of my own in the above paragraph may suggest I am immodest. That is a risk of using the first person. Yet avoiding 'I' by impersonality and circumlocution leads to dullness, and I would rather be thought conceited than dull. Articles are written to interest the reader, not to make him admire the author. Overconscientious anonymity can be overdone, as in the article by two authors which had a footnote: 'Since this article was written, unfortunately one of us has died.'

An important factor in presentation is the use of diagrams, charts, tables, and so on. I often find that I cannot understand diagrams in medical journals even when I try very hard. I take several minutes identifying the ordinates and sorting out the different types of hatching and shading and their interpretation. Then I usually find I have been looking at Fig 1 instead of Fig 2. A diagram should be used only if it makes something easier to understand. The purpose of a diagram is not to crowd as many facts as possible into the smallest space.

STYLE

Style is what matters most; grammar, syntax, spelling, and punctuation are only useful conventions. They matter very little, nor need we disapprove strongly about improper unions between Greek and Latin or we would have to say dicycle, instead of bicycle. What *does* matter is when doctors write what Ivor Brown calls 'pudder' and Sir Ernest Gowers calls 'gobbledygook'. They clog their meaning with muddy words and pompous prolixity; they spend little time in seeking the shortest, neatest, and plainest way of putting down their meaning. Quiller-Couch, A. P. Herbert, Ivor Brown, and Sir Ernest Gowers have done a great deal to encourage good writing, but I think Sir Ernest Gowers's *Plain Words* is the best of all. Unfortunately, those who need it most read it least, because anyone taking trouble to buy a book about using English will probably take trouble in writing it: style is largely a matter of taking trouble, though many people wrongly regard it as a gift. The people who write badly do not seem to realize they do, and so do not buy this admirable book.

Here is a sentence from a medical journal:

> Experiments are described which demonstrate that in normal individuals the lowest concentration in which sucrose can be detected by means of gustation differs from the lowest concentration in which sucrose (in the amount employed) has to be ingested in order to produce a demonstrable decrease in olfactory acuity and a noteworthy conversion of sensations interpreted as a satiety associated with ingestion of food.

All the author meant was: experiments are described which show that normal people can taste sugar in water in quantities not strong enough to interfere with their sense of smell or take away their appetite.

Lastly, length. Medical articles should, like after dinner speeches, finish before the audience's interest has started to wane. I finish now, pointing out that this paper, like the talk on which it is based, is intended only to provoke discussion. It solves no problems; it only poses them. It is incomplete, inaccurate, and probably irritating; but I hope—and I have spent many hours trying to achieve that end— that it is not dull.

(From *British Medical Journal*, 23 August 1958)

⇥8⇤

Ethics and Purpose

*E*THICS *have been integral to medical practice since the ancient Greeks, but for many centuries they were delivered exclusively in the form of codes. Codes are still being produced, but nowadays the precepts of codes are supplemented by ethical argument. But good ethical arguments are not the same as traditional slogans and this emerges when we see them used in the comic context of the reluctant cannibal.*

The most important ethical ideas in Greek medicine concern the need to be a competent physician and to know the limits of competence. In other words, the patient must not be harmed. These ideas reflect the fact that for the Greeks the physician had a skill (a technē), like the carpenter or the sea captain, and to be ethical was to be able to exercise that skill competently, and to know its limitations. Physicians in subsequent centuries have been required to be compassionate or beneficent, to be just, to respect the patient's autonomy, to make good use of scarce resources, and even to grapple with the meaning of life and death. Perhaps they should try to do all these things, but first they must be competent and not cause harm by attempting what they are not able to do. In that respect the virtue of the craftsman should remain the fundamental virtue of the doctor, physician as well as surgeon. This virtue is not simply one of technique; it is an ethical virtue as well. The extract, from Zen and the Art of Motorcycle Maintenance, *has been chosen to illustrate this: '. . . there is no manual that deals with the* **real** *business of motorcycle maintenance, the most important aspect of all. Caring about what you are doing . . .'*

In the Christian era, the competent doctor had also to become compassionate or beneficent, and this virtue became the one most stressed as characteristic of the good doctor. 'Caring about what you are doing' was enlarged to include 'caring about the patient to whom you are doing it'. The tension between innate compassion or beneficence and conventional rules of justice and property are illustrated in the dilemma faced by Huckleberry Finn when his conscience, saturated in the rules of the slave-owning South, is in conflict with his innate compassion towards his friend Jim, a runaway slave. But beneficence can degenerate into sentimentality or just dry up. This is the theme of Miroslav Holub's poem 'Animal Rights'. The contrast between the boundless pity for dogs that cry and the total absence of pity for patients with progressive amyotrophic lateral sclerosis is well made. In other words, an ethic of compassion must be supplemented by one based on rights and duties. Jane Austen's Emma *provides an excellent discussion of the nature of duty.*

When should people be treated as autonomous, responsible agents and when should they be seen as being in the grip of psychological states or social circumstances which undermine their autonomy? This is the question which underlies the worries of Charles and of Sebastian's family in Brideshead Revisited, *and the many excuses put to Officer Krupke in* Westside Story *are all variations on the same theme.*

There was a stage in which utilitarianism would have been rejected out of hand in any account of health-care ethics. But scarcity of resources and therefore rationing have given the theory a foothold in health care. Indeed, for some writers it is the only valid way of looking at ethics. Jeremy Bentham (1794–1832) is one of the most uncompromising of the great utilitarians, but some of the shortcomings of the theory of utility are pointed out in a witty passage by a contemporary moral philosopher—Sir Geoffrey Warnock. Beware of having a simple utilitarian as your doctor!

Let us turn finally to the questions which face all human beings, but perhaps doctors and nurses more than most. What is the point of it all? Does life mean anything? The passage from Wittgenstein's Tractatus *(written 1914–18) is obscure, but at least some of his dark utterances may speak to the reader. It is interesting to compare Wittgenstein's proposition 6.521 with Mahler's letter to Bruno Walter of the same historical period. 'When I hear music—even while I am conducting—I hear quite positive answers to all my questions, and feel perfectly clear and confident. Or rather, I feel quite clearly that there are no questions.'*

John Wisdom, who was Professor of Philosophy at Cambridge, delivered his talk 'What Is There in Horse-Racing?' on the radio in 1954. Underneath the urbane surface there is some profound thought. He reminds us that we need not always look beyond the ordinary activities of life for a purpose or meaning; their meaning lies in what they are rather than in what, if anything, they bring about. 'For a game of croquet is not merely a matter of getting balls through hoops, anymore than a conversation is a matter of getting noises out of a larynx.' Yes, or a work of art is merely a matter of sounds, words, or paint; they are that, but they are also meaningful forms of human communication, and that is their point.

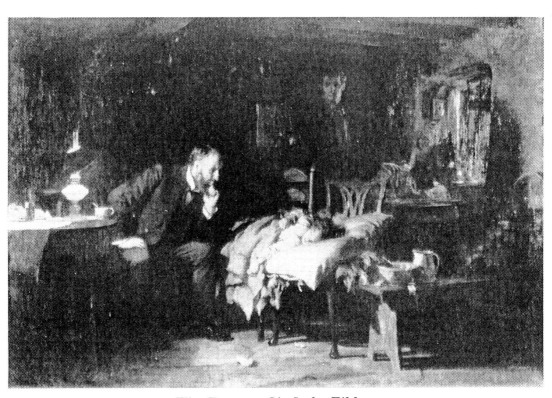

The Doctor. *Sir Luke Fildes.*
This painting is an eloquent portrayal of what medicine is all about—the doctor,
the patient, and the quality of the relationship that exists between them.
The physician is attending the patient, watching and waiting—being there.
Much of the painting's impact is in the space between the physician's eyes and the
child, which is filled, solely, by the doctor's gaze.

Ethical Argument

Michael Flanders
1922–1975
Donald Swan
1923–1994

Ethical Argument

'I WON'T eat people. Eating people is wrong.'

'It's wrong? People have always eaten people. What else is there to eat? If the ju-ju had meant us not to eat people, he wouldn't have made us of meat.'

'I don't eat people.'

'Oh no, not again!'

'I won't eat people. Eating people is wrong.'

'I never heard such a ridiculous idea in all my born days. To think that a son of mine should grow up to be a sissy. Me, chief assistant to the assistant chief! Why, if this were to get around, son, it could just about ruin me socially!'

'I won't eat people.'

'Have you been talking to one of your mothers again? I suppose you're one of these cranks that thinks it's cruel, is that it? You see a man sitting in a pot and you think he's suffering? It's not like that at all. He's just sitting there in the nice warm water, thinking of all the pleasure and happiness he's going to give to heaps of people. He knows it's better than just dying of old age. Why that man in the pot there, he enjoys it.'

'Eating people is wrong.'

'Look son, you're young. I know how you feel. I've been young myself, and when you're young you want to change the whole world over night. But it can't be done. You've got to learn to take the world as it is.'

'I won't let another man pass my lips.'

'I know why you say, "Don't eat people." Because you're a coward, that's your trouble. A yellow-livered coward. You wouldn't mind eating people if you weren't afraid of ending up in the pot yourself. You're going the right way about it too, son! They'll eat you, even if they can't digest your opinions.'

'I won't eat people.'

'Communist!'

'Don't eat people. Eating people is wrong.'

'Look, going around saying, "Don't eat people," is the way to make people hate you. People always have eaten people, always will eat people. You can't change human nature.'

'I won't eat people.'

'It must have been someone he ate.'

'I won't eat people.'

'Well I give up. He used to be a regular anthropophagus. If this crazy idealist notion of yours were to catch on, I just don't know where we'd all be. Just about ruin our entire internal economy. Fortunately its catching on isn't very likely. You might just as well say, "Don't fight people."'

(From *The Reluctant Cannibal*; wording slightly modified)

Aristotle
384–322 BC

From *Nicomachean Ethics*

BUT one thing must be agreed on from the start: the whole account of matters of conduct has to be given in outline rather than in detail, in accordance with our claim at the beginning that the accounts we look for must be appropriate to their subject-matter. Nothing is fixed in matters of conduct and of what is useful, any more than in matters of health. Since even the general account is like this, the account of particular cases is still less exact. The cases do not fall under any art or precept. Instead the agents themselves must all the time consider what is appropriate to the particular occasion, just as in medicine or navigation.

(*Translated from the Greek by Elizabeth Telfer*)

Paying Attention

Robert M. Pirsig
1928–

From *Zen and the Art of Motorcycle Maintenance*

ON an air-cooled engine like this, extreme overheating can cause a 'seizure'. This machine has had one . . . in fact, three of them. I check it from time to time the same way I would check a patient who has had a heart attack, even though it seems cured.

In a seizure, the pistons expand from too much heat, become too big for the walls of the cylinders, seize them, melt to them sometimes, and lock the engine and rear wheel and start the whole cycle into a skid. The first time this one seized, my head was pitched over the front wheel and my passenger was almost on top of me. At about thirty it freed up again and started to run but I pulled off the road and stopped to see what was wrong. All my passenger could think to say was 'What did you do *that* for?'

I shrugged and was as puzzled as he was, and stood there with the cars whizzing by, just staring. The engine was so hot the air around it shimmered and we could feel the heat radiate. When I put a wet finger on it, it sizzled like a hot iron and we rode home, slowly, with a new sound, a slap that meant the pistons no longer fit and an overhaul was needed.

I took this machine into a shop because I thought it wasn't important enough to justify getting into myself, having to learn all the complicated details and maybe having to order parts and special tools and all that time-dragging stuff when I could get someone else to do it in less time—sort of John's attitude.

The shop was a different scene from the ones I remembered. The mechanics, who had once all seemed like ancient veterans, now looked like children. A radio was going full blast and they were clowning around and talking and seemed not to notice me. When one of them finally came over he barely listened to the piston slap before saying, 'Oh yeah. Tappets.'

Tappets? I should have known then what was coming.

Two weeks later I paid their bill for 140 dollars, rode the cycle carefully at varying low speeds to wear it in and then after one thousand miles opened it up. At about seventy-five it seized again and freed at thirty, the same as before. When I brought it back they accused me of not breaking it in properly, but after much argument agreed to look into it. They overhauled it again and this time took it out themselves for a high-speed road test.

It seized on *them* this time.

After the third overhaul two months later they replaced the cylinders, put in oversize main carburetor jets, retarded the timing to make it run as coolly as possible and told me, 'Don't run it fast.'

It was covered with grease and did not start. I found the plugs were disconnected, connected them and started it, and now there really *was* a tappet noise. They hadn't adjusted them. I pointed this out and the kid came with an open-end adjustable wrench, set wrong, and swiftly rounded both of the sheet-aluminum tappet covers, ruining both of them.

'I hope we've got some more of those in stock,' he said.

I nodded.

He brought out a hammer and cold chisel and started to pound them loose. The chisel punched through the aluminum cover and I could see he was pounding the chisel right into the engine head. On the next blow he missed the chisel completely and struck the head with the hammer, breaking off a portion of two of the cooling fins.

'Just stop,' I said politely, feeling this was a bad dream. 'Just give me some new covers and I'll take it the way it is.'

I got out of there as fast as possible, noisy tappets, shot tappet covers, greasy machine, down the road, and then felt a bad vibration at speeds over twenty. At the curb I discovered two of the four engine-mounting bolts were missing and a nut was missing from the third. The whole engine was hanging on by only one bolt. The overhead-cam chain-tensioner bolt was also missing, meaning it would have been hopeless to try to adjust the tappets anyway. Nightmare.

The thought of John putting his BMW into the hands of one of those people is something I have never brought up with him. Maybe I should.

I found the cause of the seizures a few weeks later, waiting to happen again. It was a little twenty-five-cent pin in the internal oil-delivery system that had been sheared and was preventing oil from reaching the head at high speeds.

The question *why* comes back again and again and has become a major reason for wanting to deliver this Chautauqua. Why did they butcher it so? These were not people running away from technology, like John and Sylvia. These were the technologists themselves. They sat down to do a job and they performed it like chimpanzees. Nothing personal in it. There was no obvious reason for it. And I tried to think back into that shop, that nightmare place, to try to remember anything that could have been the cause.

The radio was a clue. You can't really think hard about what you're doing and listen to the radio at the same time. Maybe they didn't see their job as having anything to do with hard thought just wrench twiddling. If you can twiddle wrenches while listening to the radio that's more enjoyable.

Their speed was another clue. They were really slopping things around in a hurry and not looking where they slopped them. More money that way—if you don't stop to think that it usually takes longer or comes out worse.

But the biggest clue seemed to be their expressions. They were hard to explain. Good-natured, friendly, easygoing—and uninvolved. They were like spectators. You had the feeling they had just wandered in there themselves and somebody had handed them a wrench. There was no identification with the job. No saying, 'I am a mechanic.' At 5 p.m. or whenever their eight hours were in, you knew they would cut it off and not have another thought about their work. They were already trying not to have any thoughts about their work *on* the job. In their own way they were achieving the same thing John and Sylvia were, living with technology without really having anything to do with it. Or rather, they had something to do with it, but their own selves were outside of it, detached, removed. They were involved in it but not in such a way as to care.

Not only did these mechanics not find that sheared pin, but it was clearly a mechanic who had sheared it in the first place, by assembling the side cover plate improperly. I remembered the previous owner had said a mechanic had told him the plate was hard to get on. That was why. The shop manual had warned about this, but like the others he was probably in too much of a hurry or he didn't care.

While at work I was thinking about this same lack of care in the digital computer manuals I was editing. Writing and editing technical manuals is what I do for a living the other eleven months of the year and I knew they were full of errors, ambiguities, omissions and information so completely screwed up you had to read them six times to make any sense out of them. But what struck me for the first time was the agreement of these manuals with the spectator attitude I had seen in the shop. These were spectator manuals. It was built into the format of them. Implicit in every line is the idea that 'Here is the machine, isolated in time and in space from everything else in the universe. It has no relationship to you, you have no relationship to it, other than to turn certain switches, maintain voltage levels, check for error conditions . . .' and so on. That's it. The mechanics in their attitude toward the machine were really taking no different attitude from the manual's toward the machine, or from the attitude I had when I brought it in there. We were all spectators. And it occurred to me there *is* no manual that deals with the *real* business of motorcycle maintenance, the most important aspect of all. Caring about what you are doing is considered either unimportant or taken for granted.

On this trip I think we should notice it, explore it a little, to see if in that strange separation of what man is from what man does we may have some clues as to what the hell has gone wrong in this twentieth century. I don't want to hurry it. That itself is a poisonous twentieth-century attitude. When you want to hurry something, that means you no longer care about it and want to get on to other things. I just want to get at it slowly, but carefully and thoroughly, with the same attitude I remember was present just before I found that sheared pin. It was that attitude that found it, nothing else.

Compassion and Duty

Mark Twain
1835–1910

From *Huckleberry Finn*

J<small>IM</small> said it made him all over trembly and feverish to be so close to freedom. Well, I can tell you it made me all over trembly and feverish, too, to hear him, because I begun to get it through my head that he *was* most free—and who was to blame for it? Why, *me*. I couldn't get that out of my conscience, no how nor no way. It got to troubling me so I couldn't rest; I couldn't stay still in one place. It hadn't ever come home to me before, what this thing was that I was doing. But now it did; and it staid with me, and scorched me more and more. I tried to make out to myself that *I* warn't to blame, because *I* didn't run Jim off from his rightful owner; but it warn't no use, conscience up and says, every time, 'But you knowed he was running for his freedom, and you could a paddled ashore and told somebody.' That was so—I couldn't get around that, no way. That was where it pinched. Conscience says to me, 'What had poor Miss Watson done to you, that you could see her nigger go off right under your eyes and never say one single word? What did that poor old woman do to you, that you could treat her so mean? Why, she tried to learn you your book, she tried to learn you your manners, she tried to be good to you every way she knowed how. *That's* what she done.'

I got to feeling so mean and so miserable I most wished I was dead. I fidgeted up and down the raft, abusing myself to myself, and Jim was fidgeting up and down past me. We neither of us could keep still. Every time he danced around and says, 'Dah's Cairo!' it went through me like a shot, and I thought if it *was* Cairo I reckoned I would die of miserableness.

Jim talked out loud all the time while I was talking to myself. He was saying how the first thing he would do when he got to a free State he would go to saving up money and never spend a single cent, and when he got enough he would buy his wife, which was owned on a farm close to where Miss Watson lived; and then they would both work to buy the two children, and if their master wouldn't sell them, they'd get an Ab'litionist to go and steal them.

It most froze me to hear such talk. He wouldn't ever dared to talk such talk in his life before. Just see what a difference it made in him the minute he judged he was about free. It was according to the old saying, 'Give a nigger an inch and he'll take an ell.' Thinks I, this is what comes of my not thinking. Here was this nigger which I had as good as helped to run away, coming right out flat-footed and saying he would steal his children—children that belonged to a man I didn't even know; a man that hadn't ever done me no harm.

I was sorry to hear Jim say that, it was such a lowering of him. My conscience got to stirring me up hotter than ever, until at last I says to it, 'Let up on me—it ain't too late, yet—I'll paddle ashore at the first light, and tell.' I felt easy, and happy, and light as a feather, right off. All my troubles was gone. I went to looking out sharp for a light, and sort of singing to myself. By-and-by one showed. Jim sings out:

'We's safe, Huck, we's safe! Jump up and crack yo' heels, dat's de good ole Cairo at las', I jis knows it!'

I says:

'I'll take the canoe and go see, Jim. It mightn't be, you know.'

He jumped and got the canoe ready, and put his old coat in the bottom for me to set on, and give me the paddle; and as I shoved off, he says:

'Pooty soon I'll be a-shout'n for joy, en I'll say, it's all on accounts o' Huck; I's a free man, en I couldn't ever ben free ef it hadn' ben for Huck; Huck done it. Jim won't ever forgit you, Huck; you's de bes' fren' Jim's ever had; en you's de *only* fren' old Jim's got now.'

I was paddling off, all in a sweat to tell on him; but when he says this, it seemed to kind of take the tuck all out of me. I went along slow then, and I warn't right down certain whether I was glad I started or whether I warn't. When I was fifty yards off, Jim says:

'Dah you goes, de ole true Huck; de on'y white genlman dat ever kep' his promise to ole Jim.'

Well, I just felt sick. But I says, I *got* to do it—I can't get *out* of it. Right then, along comes a skiff with two men in it, with guns, and they stopped and I stopped. One of them says:

'What's that, yonder?'

'A piece of a raft,' I says.

'Do you belong on it?'

'Yes, sir.'

'Any men on it?'

'Only one, sir.'

'Well, there's five niggers run off tonight, up yonder above the head of the bend. Is your man white or black?'

I didn't answer up prompt. I tried to, but the words wouldn't come. I tried, for a second or two, to brace up and out with it, but I warn't man enough—hadn't the spunk of a rabbit. I see I was weakening; so I just give up trying, and up and says'

'We's white.'

'I reckon we'll go and see for ourselves.'

'I wish you would,' says I, 'because it's pap that's there, and maybe you'd help me tow the raft ashore where the light is. He's sick—and so is mam and Mary Ann.'

'Oh, the devil! we're in a hurry, boy. But I s'pose we've go to. Come—buckle to your paddle, and let's get along.'

I buckled to my paddle and they laid to their oars. When we had made a stroke or two, I says:

'Pap'll be mighty much obleeged to you, I can tell you. Everybody goes away when I want them to help me tow the raft ashore, and I can't do it by myself.'

'Well, that's infernal mean. Odd, too. Say, boy, what's the matter with your father?'

'It's the——the—well, it ain't anything much.'

They stopped pulling. It warn't but a mighty ways to the raft, now. One says:

'Boy, that's a lie. What *is* the matter with your pap? Answer up square, now, and it'll be the better for you.'

'I will, sir, I will, honest—but don't leave us, please. It's the—the—gentlemen, if you'll only pull ahead, and let me heave you the headline, you won't have to come a-near the raft—please do.'

'Set her back, John, set her back!' says one. They backed water. 'Keep away, boy—keep to looard. Confound it, I just expect the wind has blowed it to us. Your pap's got the smallpox, and you know it precious well. Why didn't you come out and say so? Do you want to spread it all over?'

'Well,' says I, a-blubbering, 'I've told everybody before, and then they just went away and left us.'

'Poor devil, there's something in that. We are right down sorry for you, but we—well, hang it, we don't want the smallpox, you see. Look here, I'll tell you what to do. Don't you try to land by yourself, or you'll smash everything to pieces. You float along down about twenty miles and you'll come to a town on the left-hand side of the river. It will be long after sun-up, then, and when you ask for help, you tell them your folks are all down with chills and fever. Don't be a fool again, and let people guess what is the matter. Now we're trying to do you a kindness; so you just put twenty miles between us, that's a good boy. It wouldn't do any good to land yonder where the light is—it's only a wood-yard. Say—I reckon your father's poor, and I'm bound to say he's in pretty hard luck. Here—I'll put a twenty dollar gold piece on this board, and you get it when it floats by. I feel mighty mean to leave you, but my kingdom! it won't do to fool with smallpox, don't you see?'

'Hold on, Parker,' says the other man, 'here's a twenty to put on the board for me. Good-bye, boy, you do as Mr Parker told you, and you'll be all right.'

'That's so, my boy—good-bye, good-bye. If you see any runaway niggers, you get help and nab them, and you can make some money by it.'

'Good-bye, sir,' says I, 'I won't let no runaway niggers get by me if I can help it.'

They went off and I got aboard the raft, feeling bad and low, because I knowed very well I had done wrong, and I see it warn't no use for me to try to learn to do right; a body that don't get *started* right when he's little, ain't got no show—when the pinch comes there ain't nothing to back him up and keep him to his work, and so he gets beat. Then I thought a minute, and says to myself, hold on,—s'pose you'd a done right and give Jim up; would you felt better than what you do now? No, says I, I'd feel bad—I'd feel just the same way I do now. Well, then, says I, what's the use you learning to do right, when it's troublesome to do right and ain't no trouble to do wrong, and the wages is just the same? I was stuck. I couldn't answer that. So I reckoned I wouldn't bother no more about it, but after this always do whichever come handiest at the time.

I went into the wigwam; Jim warn't there. I looked all around; he warn't anywhere. I says:

'Jim!'

'Here I is, Huck. Is dey out o' sight yit? Don't talk loud.'

He was in the river, under the stern oar, with just his nose out. I told him they was out of sight, so he come aboard. He says:

'I was a-listenin' to all de talk, en I slips into de river en was gwyne to shove for sho' if dey come aboard. Den I was gwyne to swim to de raf' agin when dey was gone. But lawsy, how you did fool 'em, Huck! Dat *wuz* de smartes' dodge! I tell you, chile, I 'speck it save' ole Jim—ole Jim ain't gwyne to forgit you for dat, honey.'

Miroslav Holub
1923–

Animal Rights

PITY for dogs
                 that cry
(boundless pity).
Pity for mice
                 that squirm.
Pity for earthworms
                 that wither helplessly
(limited pity)
(Pity for protozoons
                 that sway their cilia
                 so desperately.
Pity for cells
                 that crawl away
                 for life).

Pity for the central nervous system,
                 microglia excepted.

Patients
with progressive amyotrophic lateral sclerosis can just
   fuck off. They shouldn't have been born.
Hieronymus Bosch be with them
for ever and ever amen.

(*Translated from the Czech by David Young and Dana*
Hábová)

Jane Austen
1775–1817

From *Emma*

[*Editor's Note*: To appreciate the full flavour of this passage the reader should recall that Frank Churchill is Mr Weston's *son*, brought up by an aunt and uncle on his mother's death, and taking their name on his coming of age. Mr Weston has recently married again and everyone thinks that Frank should visit his father and new stepmother. It is also relevant that Mr Knightley is in love with Emma although neither of them is aware of this at this point.]

[*Chapter 18*]

MR FRANK CHURCHILL did not come. When the time proposed drew near, Mrs Weston's fears were justified in the arrival of a letter of excuse. For the present, he could not be spared, to his 'very great mortification and regret: but still he looked forward with the hope of coming to Randalls at no distant period'.

Mrs Weston was exceedingly disappointed—much more disappointed, in fact, than her husband, though her dependence on seeing the young man had been so much more sober: but a sanguine temper, though for ever expecting more good than occurs, does not always pay for its hopes by any proportionate depression. It soon flies over the present failure and begins to hope again. For half an hour Mr Weston was surprised and sorry; but then he began to perceive that Frank's coming two or three months later would be a much better plan; better time of year; better weather; and that he would be able, without any doubt, to stay considerably longer with them than if he had come sooner.

These feelings rapidly restored his comfort, while Mrs Weston, of a more apprehensive disposition, foresaw nothing but a repetition of excuses and delays; and after all her concern for what her husband was to suffer, suffered a great deal more herself.

Emma was not at this time in a state of spirits to care really about Mr Frank Churchill's not coming, except as a disappointment at Randalls. The acquaintance at present had no charm for her. She wanted, rather, to be quiet, and out of temptation; but still, as it was desirable that she should appear, in general, like her usual self, she took care to express as much interest in the circumstance, and enter as warmly into Mr and Mrs Weston's disappointment, as might naturally belong to their friendship.

She was the first to announce it to Mr Knightley: and exclaimed quite as much as was necessary (or, being acting a part, perhaps rather more) at the conduct of the Churchills, in keeping him away. She then proceeded to say a good deal more than she felt, of the advantage of such an addition to their confined society in Surrey; the pleasure of looking at somebody new; the gala-day to Highbury entire, which the sight of him would have made; and ending with reflections on the Churchills again, found herself directly involved in a disagreement with Mr Knightley: and, to her great amusement, perceived that she was taking the other side of the question from her real opinion, and making use of Mrs Weston's arguments against herself.

'The Churchills are very likely in fault,' said Mr Knightley, coolly: 'but I dare say he might come if he would.'

'I do not know why you should say so. He wishes exceedingly to come; but his uncle and aunt will not spare him.'

'I cannot believe that he has not the power of coming, if he made a point of it. It is too unlikely, for me to believe it without proof.'

'How odd you are! What has Mr Frank Churchill done, to make you suppose him such an unnatural creature?'

'I am not supposing him at all an unnatural creature, in suspecting that he may have learnt to be above his connections, and to care very little for anything but his own pleasure, from living with those who have always set him the example of it. It is a great deal more natural than one could wish, that a young man, brought up by those who are proud, luxurious, and selfish, should be proud, luxurious, and selfish too. If Frank Churchill had wanted to see his father, he would have contrived it between September and January. A man at his age—what is he?—three or four-and-twenty—cannot be without the means of doing as much as that. It is impossible.'

'That's easily said, and easily felt by you, who have always been your own master. You are the worst judge in the world, Mr Knightley, of the difficulties of dependence. You do not know what it is to have tempers to manage.'

'It is not to be conceived that a man of three or four-and-twenty should not have liberty of mind or limb to that amount. He cannot want money—he cannot want leisure. We know, on the contrary, that he has so much of both, that he is glad to get rid of them at the idlest haunts in the kingdom. We hear of him for ever at some watering-place or other. A little while ago, he was at Weymouth. This proves that he can leave the Churchills.'

'Yes, sometimes he can.'

'And those times are, whenever he thinks it worth his while; whenever there is any temptation of pleasure.'

'It is very unfair to judge of anybody's conduct, without an intimate knowledge of their situation. Nobody, who has not been in the interior of a family, can say what the difficulties of any individual of that family may be. We ought to be acquainted with Enscombe, and with Mrs Churchill's temper, before we pretend to decide upon what her nephew can do. He may, at times, be able to do a great deal more than he can at others.'

'There is one thing, Emma, which a man can always do, if he chooses, and that is, his duty; not by manœuvring and finessing, but by vigour and resolution. It is Frank Churchill's duty to pay this attention to his father. He knows it to be so, by his promises and messages; but if he wished to do it, it might be done. A man who felt rightly would say at once, simply and resolutely, to Mrs Churchill—"Every sacrifice of mere pleasure you will always find me ready to make to your convenience; but I must go and see my father immediately. I know he would be hurt by my failing in such a remark of respect to him on the present occasion. I shall, therefore, set off tomorrow."—If he would say so to her at once, in the tone of decision becoming a man, there would be no opposition made to his going.'

'No,' said Emma laughing; 'but perhaps there might be some made to his coming back again. Such language for a young man entirely dependent, to use!—Nobody but you, Mr Knightley, would imagine it possible. But you have not an idea of what is requisite in situations directly opposite to your own. Mr Frank Churchill to be making such a speech as that to the uncle and aunt, who have brought him up, and are to provide for him!—Standing up in the middle of the room, I suppose, and speaking as loud as he could!—How can you imagine such conduct practicable?'

'Depend upon it, Emma, a sensible man would find no difficulty in it. He would feel himself in the right; and the declaration—made, of course, as a man of sense would make it, in a proper manner—would do him more good, raise him higher, fix his interest stronger with the people he depended on, than all that a line of shifts and expedients can ever do. Respect would be added to affection. They would feel that they could trust him; that the nephew, who had done rightly by his father, would do rightly by them; for they know, as well as he does, as well as all the world must know, that he ought to pay this visit to his father; and while meanly exerting their power to delay it, are in their hearts not thinking the better of him for submitting to their whims. Respect for right conduct is felt by everybody. If he would act in this sort of manner, on principle, consistently, regularly, their little minds would bend to his.'

'I rather doubt that. You are very fond of bending little minds; but where little minds belong to rich people in authority, I think they have a knack of swelling out, till they are quite as unmanageable as great ones. I can imagine that if you, as you are, Mr Knightley, were to be transported and placed all at once in Mr Frank Churchill's situation, you would be able to say and do just what you have been recommending for him; and it might have a very good effect. The Churchills might not have a word to say in return; but then, you would have no habits of early obedience and long observance to break through. To him who has, it might not be so easy to burst forth at once into perfect independence, and set all their claims on his gratitude and regard at nought. He may have as strong a sense of what would be right, as you can have, without being so equal under particular circumstances to act up to it.'

'Then, it would not be so strong a sense. If it failed to produce equal exertion, it could not be an equal conviction.'

'Oh! the difference of situation and habit! I wish you would try to understand what an amiable young man may be likely to feel in directly opposing those, whom as child and boy he has been looking up to all his life.'

'Your amiable young man is a very weak young man, if this be the first occasion of his carrying through a resolution to do right against the will of others. It ought to have been an habit with him by this time, of following his duty, instead of consulting expediency. I can allow for the fears of the child, but not of the man. As he became rational, he ought to have roused himself and shaken off all that was unworthy in their authority. He ought to have opposed the first attempt on their side to make him slight his father. Had he begun as he ought, there would have been no difficulty now.'

'We shall never agree about him.' cried Emma; 'but that is nothing extraordinary. I have not the least idea of his being a weak young man: I feel sure that he is not. Mr Weston would not be blind to folly, though in his own son: but he is very likely to have a more yielding, complying, mild disposition than would suit your notions of man's perfection. I dare say he has: and though it may cut him off from some advantages, it will secure him many others.'

'Yes; all the advantages of sitting still when he ought to move, and of leading a life of mere idle pleasure, and fancying himself extremely expert in finding excuses for it. He can sit down and write a fine flourishing letter, full of professions and falsehoods, and persuade himself that he has hit upon the very best method in the world of preserving peace at home and preventing his father's having any right to complain. His letters disgust me.'

'Your feelings are singular. They seem to satisfy everybody else.'

'I suspect they do not satisfy Mrs Weston. They hardly can satisfy a woman of her good sense and quick feelings: standing in a mother's place, but without a mother's affection to blind her. It is on her account that attention to Randalls is doubly due, and she must doubly feel the omission. Had she been a person of consequence herself, he would have come I dare say; and it would not have signified whether he did or no. Can you think your friend behind-hand in these sort of considerations; Do you suppose she does not often say all this to herself? No, Emma, your amiable young man can be amiable only in French, not in English. He may be very 'aimable', have very good manners, and be very agreeable; but he can have no English delicacy towards the feelings of other people: nothing really amiable about him.'

'You seem determined to think ill of him.'

'Me!—not at all,' replied Mr Knightley, rather displeased; 'I do not want to think ill of him. I should be as ready to acknowledge his merits as any other man; but I hear of none, except what are merely personal; that he is well grown and good-looking, with smooth, plausible manners.'

'Well, if he have nothing else to recommend him, he will be a treasure at Highbury. We do not often look upon fine young men, well-bred and agreeable. We must not be nice and ask for all the virtues into the bargain. Cannot you imagine, Mr Knightley, what a *sensation* his coming will produce? There will be but one subject throughout the parishes of Donwell and Highbury; but one interest—one object of curiosity; it will be all Mr Frank Churchill; we shall think and speak of nobody else.'

'You will excuse my being so much overpowered. If I find him conversible, I shall be glad of his acquaintance; but if he is only a chattering coxcomb, he will not occupy much of my time or thoughts.'

'My idea of him is, that he can adapt his conversation to the taste of everybody, and has the power as well as the wish of being universally agreeable. To you, he will talk of farming; to me, of drawing or music; and so on to everybody, having that general information on all subjects which will enable him to follow the lead, or take the lead, just as propriety may require, and to speak extremely well on each; that is my idea of him.'

'And mine,' said Mr Knightley warmly, 'is, that if he turn out anything like it, he will be the most insufferable fellow breathing! What! at three-and-twenty to be the king of his company—the great man—the practised politician, who is to read everybody's character, and make everybody's talents conduce to the display of his own superiority; to be dispensing his flatteries around, that he may make all appear like fools compared with himself! My dear Emma, your own good sense could not endure such a puppy when it came to the point.'

'I will say no more about him,' cried Emma, 'you turn everything to evil. We are both prejudiced; you against, I for him; and we have no chance of agreeing till he is really here.'

'Prejudiced! I am not prejudiced.'

'But I am very much, and without being at all ashamed of it. My love for Mr and Mrs Weston gives me a decided prejudice in his favour.'

'He is a person I never think of from one month's end to another,' said Mr Knightley, with a degree of vexation, which made Emma immediately talk of something else, though she could not comprehend why he should be angry.

To take a dislike to a young man, only because he appeared to be of a different disposition from himself, was unworthy of the real liberality of mind which she was always used to acknowledge in him; for with all the high opinion of himself, which she had often laid to his charge, she had never before for a moment supposed it could make him unjust to the merit of another.

Evelyn Waugh
1903–1966

From *Brideshead Revisited*

THEN, back at Oxford, we took up again the life that seemed to be shrinking in the cold air. The sadness that had been strong in Sebastian the term before gave place to a kind of sullenness even towards me. He was sick at heart somewhere, I did not know how, and I grieved for him, unable to help.

When he was gay now it was usually because he was drunk, and when drunk he developed an obsession of 'mocking Mr Samgrass'. He composed a ditty of which the refrain was, 'Green arse, Samgrass—Samgrass green arse', sung to the tune of St Mary's chime, and he would thus serenade him, perhaps once a week, under his windows. Mr Samgrass was distinguished as being the first don to have a private telephone installed in his rooms. Sebastian in his cups used to ring him up and sing him this simple song. And all this Mr Samgrass took in good part, as it is called, smiling obsequiously when we met, but with growing confidence, as though each outrage in some way strengthened his hold on Sebastian.

It was during this term that I began to realize that Sebastian was a drunkard in quite a different sense to myself. I got drunk often, but through an excess of high spirits, in the love of the moment, and the wish to prolong and enhance it; Sebastian drank to escape. As we together grew older and more serious I drank less, he more. I found that sometimes after I had gone back to my college, he sat up late and alone, soaking. A succession of disasters came on him so swiftly and with such unexpected violence that it is hard to say when exactly I recognized that my friend was in deep trouble. I knew it well enough in the Easter vacation.

Julia used to say, 'Poor Sebastian. It's something chemical in him.'

That was the cant phrase of the time, derived from heaven knows what misconception of popular science. 'There's something chemical between them' was used to explain the over-mastering hate or love of any two people. It was the old concept of determinism in a new form. I do not believe there was anything chemical in my friend.

The Easter party at Brideshead was a bitter time, culminating in a small but unforgettably painful incident. Sebastian got very drunk before dinner in his mother's house, and thus marked the beginning of a new epoch in his melancholy record, another stride in the flight from his family which brought him to ruin.

It was at the end of the day when the large Easter party left Brideshead. It was called the Easter party, though in fact it began on the Tuesday of Easter Week, for the Flytes all went into retreat at the guest-house of a monastery from Maundy Thursday until Easter. This year Sebastian had said he would not go, but at the last moment had yielded, and came home in a state of acute depression from which I totally failed to raise him.

He had been drinking very hard for a week—only I knew how hard—and drinking in a nervous, surreptitious way, totally unlike his old habit. During the party there was always a grog tray in the library, and Sebastian took to slipping in there at odd moments during the day without saying anything even to me. The house was largely deserted during the day. I was at work painting another panel in the little garden-room in the colonnade. Sebastian complained of a cold, stayed in, and during all that time was never quite sober; he escaped attention by being silent. Now and then I noticed him attract curious glances, but most of the party knew him too slightly to see the change in him, while his own family were occupied, each with their particular guests.

When I remonstrated he said, 'I can't stand all these people about,' but it was when they finally left and he had to face his family at close quarters that he broke down.

The normal practice was for a cocktail tray to be brought into the drawing-room at six; we mixed our own drinks and the bottles were removed when we went to dress; later, just before dinner, cocktails appeared again, this time handed round by the footmen.

Sebastian disappeared after tea; the light had gone and I spent the next hour playing mah-jong with Cordelia. At six I was alone in the drawing-room, when he returned; he was frowning in a way I knew all too well, and when he spoke I recognized the drunken thickening in his voice.

'Haven't they brought the cocktails yet?' He pulled clumsily on the bell-rope.

I said, 'Where have you been?'

'Up with nanny.'

'I don't believe it. You've been drinking somewhere.'

'I've been reading in my room. My cold's worse today'.

When the tray arrived he slopped gin and vermouth into a tumbler and carried it out of the room with him. I followed him upstairs, where he shut his bedroom door in my face and turned the key.

I returned to the drawing-room full of dismay and foreboding.

The family assembled. Lady Marchmain said: 'What's become of Sebastian?'

'He's gone to lie down. His cold is worse.'

'Oh dear, I hope he isn't getting flu. I thought he had a feverish look once or twice lately. Is there anything he wants?'

'No, he particularly asked not to be disturbed.'

I wondered whether I ought to speak to Brideshead, but that grim, rock-crystal mask forbade all confidence. Instead, on the way upstairs to dress, I told Julia.

'Sebastian's drunk.'

'He can't be. He didn't even come for a cocktail.'

'He's been drinking in his room all the afternoon.'

'How very peculiar! What a bore he is! Will he be all right for dinner?'

'No.'

'Well, *you* must deal with him. It's no business of mine. Does he often do this?'

'He has lately.'

'How very boring.'

I tried Sebastian's door, found it locked, and hoped he was sleeping, but, when I came back from my bath, I found him sitting in the chair before my fire; he was dressed for dinner, all but his shoes, but his tie was awry and his hair on end; he was very red in the face and squinting slightly. He spoke indistinctly.

'Charles, what you said was quite true. Not with nanny. Been drinking whisky up here. None in the library now party's gone. Now party's gone and only mummy. Feeling rather drunk. Think I'd better have something-on-a-tray up here. Not dinner with mummy.'

'Go to bed,' I told him. 'I'll say your cold's worse.'

'Much worse.'

I took him to his room which was next to mine and tried to get him to bed, but he sat in front of his dressing-table squinnying at himself in the glass, trying to remake his bow-tie. On the writing-table by the fire was a half-empty decanter of whisky. I took it up, thinking he would not see, but he spun round from the mirror and said: 'You put that down.'

'Don't be an ass, Sebastian. You've had enough.'

'What the devil's it got to do with you? You're only a guest here—*my* guest. I drink what I want to in my own house.'

He would have fought me for it at that moment.

'Very well,' I said, putting the decanter back, 'only for God's sake keep out of sight.'

'Oh, mind your own business. You came here as my friend; now you're spying on me for my mother, I know. Well, you can get out, and tell her from me that I'll choose my friends and she her spies in future.'

So I left him and went down to dinner.

'I've been in to Sebastian,' I said. 'His cold has come on rather badly. He's gone to bed and says he doesn't want anything.'

'Poor Sebastian,' said Lady Marchmain. 'He'd better have a glass of hot whisky. I'll go and have a look at him.'

'Don't mummy, I'll go,' said Julia rising.

'*I'll* go,' said Cordelia, who was dining down that night, for a treat to celebrate the departure of the guests. She was at the door and through it before anyone could stop her.

Julia caught my eye and gave a tiny, sad shrug.

In a few minutes Cordelia was back, looking grave. 'No, he doesn't seem to want anything,' she said.

'How was he?'

'Well, I don't *know*, but I *think* he's very drunk,' she said.

'*Cordelia.*'

Suddenly the child began to giggle. ' "Marquis's Son Unused to Wine",' she quoted. ' "Model Student's Career Threatened".'

'Charles, is this true?' asked Lady Marchmain.

'Yes.'

Then dinner was announced, and we went to the dining-room where the subject was not mentioned.

When Brideshead and I were left alone he said: 'Did you say Sebastian was drunk?'

'Yes.'

'Extraordinary time to choose. Couldn't you stop him?'

'No.'

'No,' said Brideshead, 'I don't suppose you could. I once saw my father drunk, in this room. I wasn't more than about ten at the time. You can't stop people if they want to get drunk. My mother couldn't stop my father, you know.'

He spoke in his odd, impersonal way. The more I saw of this family, I reflected, the more singular I found them. 'I shall ask my mother to read to us tonight.'

It was the custom, I learned later, always to ask Lady Marchmain to read aloud on evenings of family tension. She had a beautiful voice and great humour of expression. That night she read part of *The Wisdom of Father Brown*. Julia sat with a stool covered with manicure things and carefully revarnished her nails; Cordelia nursed Julia's Pekinese; Brideshead played patience; I sat unoccupied studying the pretty group they made, and mourning my friend upstairs.

But the horrors of that evening were not yet over.

It was sometimes Lady Marchmain's practice, when the family were alone, to visit the chapel before going to bed. She had just closed her book and proposed going there when the door opened and Sebastian appeared. He was dressed as I had last seen him, but now instead of being flushed he was deathly pale.

'Come to apologize,' he said.

'Sebastian, dear, do go back to your room,' said Lady Marchmain. 'We can talk about it in the morning.'

'Not to you. Come to apologize to Charles. I was bloody to him and he's my guest. He's my guest and my only friend and I was bloody to him.'

A chill spread over us. I led him back to his room; his family went to their prayers. I noticed when we got upstairs that the decanter was now empty. 'It's time you were in bed,' I said.

Sebastian began to weep. 'Why do you take their side against me? I knew you would if I let you meet them. Why do you spy on me?'

He said more than I can bear to remember, even at twenty years' distance. At last I got him to sleep and very sadly went to bed myself.

It was touching to see the faith which everybody put in the value of a day's hunting. Lady Marchmain, who looked in on me during the morning, mocked herself for it with that delicate irony for which she was famous.

'I've always detested hunting,' she said, 'because it seems to produce a particularly gross kind of caddishness in the nicest people. I don't know what it is, but the moment they dress up and get on a horse they become like a lot of Prussians. And so boastful after it. The evenings I've sat at dinner appalled at seeing the men and women I know, transformed into half-awake, self-opinionated, mono-maniac louts! . . . and yet, you know—it must be something derived from centuries ago—my heart is quite light today to think of Sebastian out with them. "There's nothing wrong with him really," I say, "he's gone hunting"—as though it were an answer to prayer.'

She asked me about my life in Paris. I told her of my rooms with their view of the river and the towers of Notre Dame. 'I'm hoping Sebastian will come and stay with me when I go back.'

'It would have been lovely,' said Lady Marchmain, sighing as though for the unattainable.

'I hope he's coming to stay with me in London.'

'Charles, you know it isn't possible. London's the worst place. Even Mr Samgrass couldn't hold him there. We have no secrets in this house. He was *lost*, you know, all through Christmas. Mr Samgrass only found him because he couldn't pay his bill in the place where he was, so they telephoned our house. It's too horrible. No, London is impossible; if he can't behave himself here, with us. . . . We must keep him happy and healthy here for a bit, hunting, and then send him abroad again with Mr Samgrass. . . . You see, I've been through all this before.'

The retort was there, unspoken, well-understood by both of us—'You couldn't keep *him*; *he* ran away. So will Sebastian. Because they both hate you.'

A horn and the huntsman's cry sounded in the valley below us.

'There they go now, drawing the home woods. I hope he's having a good day.'

Thus with Julia and Lady Marchmain I reached deadlock, not because we failed to understand one another, but because we understood too well. With Brideshead, who came home to luncheon and talked to me on the subject—for the subject was everywhere in the house like a fire deep in the hold of a ship, below the water-line, black and red in the darkness, coming to light in acrid wisps of smoke that oozed under hatches and billowed suddenly from the scuttles and air pipes—with Brideshead, I was in a strange world, a dead world to me, in a moon-landscape of barren lava, a high place of toiling lungs.

He said: 'I hope it is dipsomania. That is simply a great misfortune that we must all help him bear. What I used to fear was that he just got drunk deliberately when he liked and because he liked.'

'That's exactly what he did—what we both did. It's what he does with me now. I can keep him to that, if only your mother would trust me. If you worry him with keepers and cures he'll be a physical wreck in a few years.'

'There's nothing *wrong* in being a physical wreck, you know. There's no moral obligation to be Postmaster-General or Master of Foxhounds or to live to walk ten miles at eighty.'

'*Wrong*,' I said. '*Moral obligation*—now you're back on religion again.'

'I never left it,' said Brideshead.

'D'you know, Bridey, if I ever felt for a moment like becoming a Catholic, I should only have to talk to you for five minutes to be cured. You manage to reduce what seem quite sensible propositions to stark nonsense.'

'It's odd you should say that. I've heard it before from other people. It's one of the many reasons why I don't think I should make a good priest. It's something in the way my mind works, I suppose.'

Stephen Sondheim
1930–

Gee, Officer Krupke

DEAR kindly Sergeant Krupke,
You gotta understand,
It's just our bringing up-ke
That gets us out of hand.
Our mothers all are junkies.
Our fathers all are drunks.
Golly Moses, natcherly we're punks!

Gee, Officer Krupke, we're very upset;
We never had the love that ev'ry child oughta get.
We ain't no delinquents, we're misunderstood.
Deep down inside us there is good.
There is good, there is good, there is untapped good.
Like inside, the worst of us is good!

Dear kindly Judge, your Honor,
My parents treat me rough,
With all their marijuana,
They won't give me a puff.

They didn't wanna have me,
But somehow I was had.
Leapin' lizards, that's why I'm so bad!

Officer Krupke, you're really a square;
This boy don't need a judge, he needs a analyst's care!
It's just his neurosis that oughta be curbed,
He's psychologic'ly disturbed.
We're disturbed, we're disturbed, we're the most disturbed,
Like we're psychologic'ly disturbed.

My father is a bastard,
My ma's an S.O.B.,
My grandpa's always plastered,
My grandma pushes tea.
My sister wears a mustache,
My brother wears a dress.
Goodness gracious, that's why I'm a mess!

Officer Krupke, you're really a slob,
This boy don't need a doctor, just a good honest job.
Society's played him a terrible trick,
And sociologic'ly he's sick!
I am sick, we are sick, we are sick, sick, sick,
Like we're sociologic'ly sick.

Dear kindly social worker,
They say go earn a buck,
Like be a soda jerker,
Which means like be a schmuck.
It's not I'm antisocial,
I'm only anti-work.
Glory-osky, that's why I'm a jerk.

Officer Krupke, you've done it again,
This boy don't need a job, he needs a year in the pen.
It ain't just a question of misunderstood;
Deep down inside him, he's no good!
I'm no good! we're no good! we're no earthly good.
Like the best of us is no damn good!

The trouble is he's crazy,
The trouble is he drinks.
The trouble is he's lazy,
The trouble is he stinks.
The trouble is he's growing,
The trouble is he's grown!
Krupke, we got troubles of our own!

Gee, Officer Krupke, we're down on our knees,
Cause no one wants a fellow with a social disease.
Gee, officer Krupke, what are we to do?

Gee, officer Krupke, krup you!

(From Westside Story, 1956)

Utility

Ruth Richardson
1951–
Brian Hurwitz
1951–

Jeremy Bentham's Self-Image: An Exemplary Bequest for Dissection

THE eighteenth-century philosopher and law reformer Jeremy Bentham still sits above ground, in his Sunday best. He died in 1832 and, in keeping with his doctrine of Utility, left his body for dissection. He expected to gain deathbed comfort from the thought that: 'How little service soever it may have been in my power to render to mankind during my lifetime, I shall at least be not altogether useless after my death.'

But this was to be no ordinary bequest for dissection. Bentham conceived that a corpse had twofold use-value—transitory: 'anatomical, or dissectional'; and more permanent: 'conservative, or statuary'. The 'savage ingenuity' of the indigenous New Zealanders had inspired Bentham to direct that his head be dried and preserved. During his lifetime experiments were made using the oven at Bentham's own house. His skeleton was to be reassembled, fully clothed, and exhibited in a glass case. This reconstructed entity he termed his auto-icon, or self-image. For the previous 20 years the grand old man had carried in his pocket the glass eyeballs which would adorn his dehydrated head.

BODIES FOR ANATOMICAL ENQUIRY

To ensure that his plan would be adopted Bentham arranged to bequeath his body to his 'dear friend' Dr Thomas Southwood Smith, author of an influential article

'Use of the Dead to the Living', which had appeared in the *Westminster Review* in 1824. At the time anatomy was in bad repute as a result of widespread grave robbery. There existed no legal source of bodies for dissection other than those of hanged murderers. In all but the most enlightened circles, dissection was deeply feared, regarded by law since Tudor times as a fate worse than death.

Southwood Smith's theme had been the immeasurable utility of anatomical knowledge. He highlighted its value in diagnosis and treatment. An anatomical understanding of referred pain would ensure, for example, that irrelevant operations would not be attempted in cases of right shoulder tip or referred knee pain. Only by close study of 'this curious and complicated machine', the human body, could commonly performed surgery, such as amputation and hernia repair, be safely undertaken. His argument remains unanswerable:

> Disease, which it is the object of these arts to prevent and to cure, is denoted by disordered function: disordered function cannot be understood without a knowledge of healthy function; healthy function cannot be understood without a knowledge of structure; structure cannot be understood unless it be examined.

Who, then, would provide subjects for anatomical enquiry: the living or the dead, the rich or the poor? A public choice must be made: allow the dissection of the dead or accept that surgeons would otherwise be driven to obtain knowledge by practising on the bodies of the living. The social implications of adopting the latter course were stark. The rich, Southwood Smith pointed out, would always have it in their power to select experienced surgeons. Such a choice was not available to the poor. Public hospitals and poorhouses would therefore be converted 'into so many schools where the surgeon by practising on the poor would learn to operate on the rich with safety and dexterity'. In 1824 the resolution to this problem was clear to Southwood Smith: the unclaimed dead from poorhouses and hospitals must be requisitioned for dissection. 'If the dead bodies of the poor are not appropriated to this use, their living bodies will and must be.'

BENTHAM'S DECISION

Jeremy Bentham had decided to bequeath his body for dissection in 1769 when he was 21, over half a century before Southwood Smith's article. Undoubtedly, Bentham intended by his example to promote bequests for anatomy. Yet he was certainly influenced by Southwood Smith. Within two years of the publication of

'Use of the Dead to the Living', Bentham drafted legislation—which was to provide a basis for the 1832 Anatomy Act—along the very lines suggested.

In the eight years between 1824 and 1832, the climate of opinion changed. Parliament became increasingly receptive to the idea of legislation on the subject. Doctors had been convicted of receiving stolen bodies, and the proprietors of anatomy schools, all of which were then privately run, were increasingly fearful of riots. A horrifying escalation had occurred in the lengths to which illicit suppliers of anatomy schools were prepared to go to obtain their merchandise. Hitherto demand had been met, and lucrative income secured, by body-snatching from graves. But in Edinburgh Burke and Hare, and later the London 'Burkers' Bishop and Williams, were shown to have resorted to murder. Thomas Wakley of the *Lancet* referred to them as 'trading assassins' and declared it 'disgusting to talk of anatomy as a science, whilst it is cultivated by means . . . which would disgrace a nation of cannibals'.

The 1832 Anatomy Act permitted those having lawful custody of dead bodies to donate them for dissection. The masters of poorhouses and hospitals could cut expenditure on pauper funerals by donating the bodies of patients too poor to provide for their own burial. By creating a cheap, legal, and institutionalized source of bodies, the Act led to the collapse of the body-snatching trade. The Anatomy Act and the inspectorate it established are still in effect.

Although it seemed to offer a welcome end to grave robbery, the prospect of such legislation provoked strong popular opposition. Dissection had hitherto been a punishment administered by law only upon executed murderers. Now it was to be visited solely upon the destitute. Feelings were running high. In 1831–2 Great Britain was in the grip of its first ever epidemic of Asiatic cholera, which in its first year claimed over 30,000 lives. Moreover, agitation to gain franchise and parliamentary reform had generated national political ferment, which reached a climax in the Great Reform Bill of 1832. Although a huge mobilization of popular opinion had succeeded in propelling an unwilling Parliament towards reform the line for voting rights was drawn at a £10 property qualification, which effectively defined and excluded the working classes. The Reform Bill received its royal assent the day after Bentham died; the Anatomy Act followed within two months. Legislation in 1752 which had made dissection available as a punishment in all cases of murder had described dissection as a 'Terror and peculiar Mark of Infamy'. The 1832 Anatomy Act transferred this 'terror' to the voteless and destitute poor.

ORATION OVER THE CORPSE

Bentham died on 6 June 1832, while the Anatomy Bill was between its first and second readings in the Lords. Invitations were swiftly printed and distributed to a select number of followers and admirers:

> Sir,
> It was the earnest desire of the late JEREMY BENTHAM that his Body should be appropriated to an illustration of the Structure and Functions of the Human Frame. In compliance with this wish, Dr Southwood Smith will deliver a Lecture, over the Body, on the Usefulness of Knowledge of this kind to the Community. The Lecture will be delivered at the Webb-street School of Anatomy and Medicine, Webb-street, Borough, Tomorrow, at Three o'Clock; at which the honour of your presence, and that of any two friends who may wish to accompany you, is requested.
> Friday, 8th June, 1832.

Southwood Smith, a physician and non-conformist preacher, began by referring to Bentham as 'foremost among the benefactors of the human race', the Newton of social philosophy. He paid respect to the dead man's courage and to his abhorrence of the prejudice against dissection. Smith spoke tenderly of bereavement and of emotional attachment to the corpse: 'For such feelings there is a foundation in the human heart. They belong to that class of feelings which require control, and sometimes, even, sacrifice.' While he was speaking a thunderstorm broke, which shook the building. With a face 'as white as that of the dead philosopher before him' he continued in a 'clear unfaltering voice'. Bentham, he said, wished to set an example to others to rise above their prejudice. Between flashes of lightning, Southwood Smith turned full on his audience, among whom were leading political and intellectual figures, some of whom had steered the Anatomy Bill through Parliament, and asked:

> How is it to be expected that the uninstructed and ignorant . . . will sacrifice their own feelings for the public good, when the best regulated shrink from the obligation? . . . It is our duty, not by legislative enactments to force others to submit to that which we are unwilling should be done to ourselves, but to set the example of making a voluntary sacrifice for the sake of a good which we profess to understand and appreciate.

The Southwood Smith of 1832 who criticized so passionately the hypocrisy of his peers seems a different man from the one who had argued eight years earlier for a wholesale appropriation of the poorhouse dead. During this period Southwood Smith had been incubating a growing awareness of the grounds for popular opposition. The poor, he had said in 1829, 'suppose that they must still serve their masters even after death has set them free from toil, and that when the early dawn can no longer rouse them from the pallet of straw to work, they must be dragged from what should be their last bed, to show in common with the murderer, how the knife of the surgeon may best avoid the rich man's artery, and least afflict the rich man's nerve.'

Between writing 'Use of the Dead to the Living' and giving the oration over Bentham's corpse, Southwood Smith had evidently come to appreciate—and dislike—the political implications of his original suggestion. He foresaw that the coercive nature of the Anatomy Act would do nothing to lessen popular hostility to dissection. The only way to achieve this was to encourage bequests. The oration over Bentham's body was therefore the perfect occasion for Southwood Smith to expound his views. Notwithstanding the dramatic power of his oratory, few, if any, of those present would prove willing to bequeath their own bodies to science.

(The complete and fully referenced version can be found in the *British Medical Journal*, 295 (18 July 1987), 195–8)

Geoffrey Warnock
1923–
Utility

. . . SUPPOSE that I, a simple Utilitarian, entrust the care of my health to a simple Utilitarian doctor. Now I know, of course, that his intentions are generally beneficent, but equally that they are not *uniquely* beneficent towards me. Thus, while he will not malevolently kill me off, I cannot be sure that he will always try to cure me of my afflictions; I can be sure only that he will do so, *unless* his assessment of the 'general happiness' leads him to do otherwise. I cannot of course condemn this attitude, since it is the same as my own; but it is more than possible that I might not much like it, and might find myself put to much anxiety and fuss in trying to detect, at successive consultations, what his intentions actually were. But conspicuously, there are two things that I could not do to diminish my anxieties: I could not get him to promise, in the style of the Hippocratic Oath, always and only to deploy his skills to my advantage; nor could I usefully ask him to disclose his intentions. The reason is essentially the same in each case. Though he might, if I asked him to, promise not to kill me off, he would of course keep this promise only if he judged it best on the whole to do so; knowing that, I could not unquestioningly rely on his keeping it; and knowing *that*, he would realize that, since I would not do so, it would matter that much less if he did not keep it. And so on, until his 'promise' becomes perfectly idle. Similarly, if I ask him what his intentions are, he will answer truthfully only if he judges it best on the whole to do so; knowing that, I will not unqualifiedly believe him; and knowing *that*, he will realize that, since I will not do so, it will matter that much less if he professes intentions that he does not actually have. And so on, until my asking and his answering become a pure waste of breath. And this is quite general; if general felicific beneficence were the only criterion, then promising and talking alike would become wholly idle pursuits. At best, as perhaps in diplomacy, what people said would become merely a part of the evidence on the basis of which one might try to decide what they really believed, or intended, or were likely to do; and it is not always obvious that there is much point in diplomacy.

(From *The Object of Morality*, 1971)

⇥ ⇤

Purpose and Meaning

Ludwig Wittgenstein
1889–1951

The Meaning of Life as Transcendental

6.41   THE sense of the world must lie outside the world. In the world everything is as it is, and everything happens as it does happen: *in* it no value exists—and if it did exist, it would have no value.

If there is any value that does have value, it must lie outside the whole sphere of what happens and is the case. For all that happens and is the case is accidental.

What makes it non-accidental cannot lie *within* the world, since if it did it would itself be accidental.

It must lie outside the world.

6.42   And so it is impossible for there to be propositions of ethics.

Propositions can express nothing that is higher.

6.421   It is clear that ethics cannot be put into words.

Ethics is transcendental.

(Ethics and aesthetics are one and the same.)

6.422   When an ethical law of the form, 'Thou shalt . . .' is laid down, one's first thought is, 'And what if I do not do it?' It is clear, however, that ethics has nothing to do with punishment and reward in the usual sense of the terms. So our question about the *consequences* of an action must be unimportant.—At least those consequences should not be events. For there must be something right about the question we posed. There must indeed be some kind of ethical reward and ethical punishment, but they must reside in the action itself.

(And it is also clear that the reward must be something pleasant and the punishment something unpleasant.)

6.423   It is impossible to speak about the will in so far as it is the subject of ethical attributes.

And the will as a phenomenon is of interest only to psychology.

6.43   If the good or bad exercise of the will does alter the world, it can alter only the limits of the world, not the facts—not what can be expressed by means of language.

In short the effect must be that it becomes an altogether different world. It must, so to speak, wax and wane as a whole.

The world of the happy man is a different one from that of the unhappy man.

6.431   So too at death the world does not alter, but comes to an end.

6.4311   Death is not an event in life: we do not live to experience death.

If we take eternity to mean not infinite temporal duration but timelessness, then eternal life belongs to those who live in the present.

Our life has no end in just the way in which our visual field has no limits.

6.4312   Not only is there no guarantee of the temporal immortality of the human soul, that is to say of its eternal survival after death; but, in any case, this assumption completely fails to accomplish the purpose for which it has always been intended. Or is some riddle solved by my surviving for ever? Is not this eternal life itself as much of a riddle as our present life? The solution of the riddle of life in space and time lies *outside* space and time.

(It is certainly not the solution of any problems of natural science that is required.)

6.432   *How* things are in the world is a matter of complete indifference for what is higher. God does not reveal himself *in* the world.

6.4321   The facts all contribute only to setting the problem, not to its solution.

6.44   It is not *how* things are in the world that is mystical, but *that* it exists.

6.45   To view the world *sub specie aeterni* is to view it as a whole—a limited whole.

Feeling the world as a limited whole—it is this that is mystical.

6.5   When the answer cannot be put into words, neither can the question be put into words.

The riddle does not exist.

If a question can be framed at all, it is also *possible* to answer it.

6.51   Scepticism is *not* irrefutable, but obviously nonsensical, when it tries to raise doubts where no questions can be asked.

For doubt can exist only where a question exists, a question only where an answer exists, and an answer only where something *can be said*.

6.52   We feel that even when *all possible* scientific questions have been answered, the problems of life remain completely untouched. Of course there are then no questions left, and this itself is the answer.

6.521   The solution of the problem of life is seen in the vanishing of the problem.

(Is not this the reason why those who have found after a long period of doubt that the sense of life became clear to them have then been unable to say what constituted that sense?)

6.522   There are, indeed, things that cannot be put into words. They *make themselves manifest*. They are what is mystical.

6.53   The correct method in philosophy would really be the following: to say nothing except what can be said, i.e. propositions of natural science—i.e. something that has nothing to do with philosophy—and then, whenever someone else wanted to say something metaphysical, to demonstrate to him that he had failed to give a meaning to certain signs in his propositions. Although it would not be satisfying to the other person— he would not have the feeling that we were teaching him philosophy— *this* method would be the only strictly correct one.

6.54   My propositions serve as elucidations in the following way: anyone who understands me eventually recognizes them as nonsensical, when he has used them—as steps—to climb up beyond them. (He must, so to speak, throw away the ladder after he has climbed up it.)

He must transcend these propositions, and then he will see the world aright.

7   What we cannot speak about we must pass over in silence.

(From *Tractatus Logico-Philosophicas*, 1922. *Translated from the German by D. F. Pears and B. F. McGuinness*)

Gustav Mahler
1860–1911

From *a Letter to Bruno Walter*

[New York, beginning of 1909]

I HAVE so much to write about myself, that I don't know where to begin. I have been going through such a continuous process of experience (in the last eighteen months) that I can hardly find words for them.

How can I attempt to describe such a tremendous crisis! I see everything in such a new light—I am so constantly on the move; sometimes it would hardly surprise me to discover that I'd suddenly taken on a new body (like Faust in the last Scene). My thirst for life is keener than ever, and I find the 'habit of living' even sweeter than before. . . .

I find myself more unimportant with every passing day, yet often fail to understand how one can go jogging along in the old daily rut, amid all the 'sweet habits of life. . . .'

But how foolish it is to let oneself be sucked into the hurly-burly of life! To be unfaithful, even for an hour, to oneself and the higher powers above! But I am writing just at random—for at the very next opportunity, for instance now when I leave this room, I shall certainly return to being as foolish as everyone else. So what is it that *thinks* in us? And what *acts* in us?

It's a strange thing! When I hear music—even while I am conducting—I hear quite positive answers to all my questions, and feel perfectly clear and confident. Or rather, I feel quite clearly that there are no questions. . . .

(Translated from the German by Daphne Woodward)

John Wisdom
1904–1993

What Is There in Horse-Racing?

I REMEMBER walking with my nurse up the village green at home. Suddenly up the road behind us a horse and light spring cart came by. It was a farmer we knew, his name was Mr Abbot; he sat on a single board, his head sunk somewhat between his shoulders, and he looked neither to left or right. His bowler rammed well down on his head was elderly, but his horse was immaculately turned out, gleaming coat, neat mane, banged tail. What I noted with anxiety was the terrific stride with which it covered the ground. Was it faster than my father's horse? And then I was a little anxious about the pony another neighbour, Mrs Russell, used to drive. She used to drive herself, her child, and the nurse to Church on Sundays. I can hear now the clamour of the church bells as she pulls up in the rectory yard. 'Nine and a half minutes this morning, Arthur,' she says as she sweeps the traces into circles and hurries the pony into a stall, for now at any moment the bells may change to that single note which means that the parson and choir are under starter's orders.

Nine and a half minutes for two and a half miles meant then the air on your face, the slight swing and lurch of the vehicle, the rasp of wheels in the mud, and the beat of the horse's hooves as, swinging round the corners of the winding lanes, you checked him a trifle before descending a steepish pitch and now again you let him go. Recently in an aeroplane I passed over the twenty miles of the Channel in about seven minutes, but we hardly seemed to move. It was excellent in its way, but was not what we meant when we used to speak of a horse that could travel.

Travel and transport: surely it is here that man has most successfully solved his difficulties. Surely here, if anywhere, he has reached his goal. And no doubt he has done a good job. And yet here, too, there appears that exasperating feature of so much success. What you gain on the roundabouts you lose on the swings. And it is not merely that: that's the trouble—it is that, in achieving what seemed the essence of what we wanted, we find the essence has eluded us; in cutting out what seemed to hinder or to be irrelevant to our satisfaction, we find that what gives contentment is more entangled with the tiresome than we had supposed. Surely when a man sets out on a journey his goal is to reach that journey's end as fast as possible, as speedily as may be. And isn't speed a matter of passing from one point to another in the minimum of time? And yet, just as we have it all laid out so that we have only to press a button to be where we want to be, just then the whole thing is apt to seem absurd. Just then we are apt to realize that what we needed was not merely to be at our destination.

This feeling of collapse and absurdity which comes over us in so many things may come over us in a small but sharp way in the simple matter of a horse race. We have won, perhaps, and the 'all right' flags are flying, but somehow the whole thing seems ridiculous. I am not pretending that this sort of dissatisfaction is always misplaced. Not at all. We may indeed have had things out of focus. But, on the other hand, the arguments by which we confirm in ourselves or spread in others such feelings of sudden contempt or depression are often muddled. And it is interesting to notice that the same arguments by which clever persons sometimes represent to us as worthless things much bigger than horse racing are also used in this smaller matter. And here, too, they are fallacious. You know how they run. They are presented in the form of questions with an innuendo. Someone asks, or perhaps one asks oneself: 'What is the purpose of it all? What is there in it? What is it but a matter of whether one horse has his head in front of another?'

These questions have a familiar and worthy ring. They may voice a useful challenge. But they need watching. Behind the words 'What is the *purpose* of racing?' lies the innuendo that if it doesn't serve a purpose it is no good and a waste of time and absurd. But the innuendo is itself absurd. For those things, such as surgical operations, or hewing coal, or what you will, which do serve a purpose, do so only because they are means to things which are worth while in themselves, worth while not because of any purpose they serve but because of what is in them—health and well-being before a warm fire, playing with a friend a game of draughts or ludo, if you like. With some things it is easy to realize that there is more in them than meets the eye or can be put into words—music, poetry, mathematics—though even here we have the muddled critics who ask in a complaining way: 'What purpose do they serve?' However, here we may boldly answer for we have the support of the good and the great: 'These things aren't merely means, they are part of what makes our lives worth while.' With other things it is not so easy. Some things seem small, seem easy, and seem to have little in them; and then, if we give time to them, we feel bound to answer 'What is there in them?'

What is there in racing? Behind such a question is another innuendo, the innuendo that if we cannot set out in words what makes a thing worth while then it isn't worth while. But this won't do. Maybe there are no words which will do this fairly, or maybe we haven't the skill to find them. I could not say what makes 'Hamlet' a good play; perhaps I could give hints; perhaps someone more skilled than I could do better. But, however skilled he were, I am sure that much of what makes 'Hamlet' 'Hamlet' will run between his fingers, much of it anyway. And this is not less true of small things. I could not put into words what may make a game of croquet on the rectory lawn something one remembers. One may give hints. A game of croquet may have a flavour sweet or bitter. For a game of croquet is not merely a matter of getting balls through hoops, any more than a conversation is merely a matter of getting noises out of a larynx. Both in croquet and conversation, human personality finds expression; human personalities are joined whether for good or not.

⊰ ACKNOWLEDGEMENTS ⊱

Dannie Abse, from *Collected Poems,* © Dannie Abse 1989. Reprinted by permission of Sheil Land Associates Ltd.

Fleur Adcock, 'The Soho Hospital for Women', © Fleur Adcock. Reprinted by permission of Oxford University Press.

Anon., Socratic dialogue. Reprinted by permission of *The Lancet.*

Anon. translated by Arthur Waley, 'Plucking the Rushes' from *Poems from the Chinese.* Published in the USA in *Translations from the Chinese* by Arthur Waley, translator. Copyright 1919 and renewed 1947 by Arthur Waley. Reprinted by permission of Allen & Unwin, now Unwin Hyman, an imprint of HarperCollins Publishers Limited, and Alfred A. Kopf, Inc.

Richard Asher, 'Is Baldness Psychological?', © The Estate of Richard Asher (The Keynes Press, 1983); 'Why are Medical Journals so Dull?', *British Medical Journal,* 23 August 1958. © British Medical Journal 1958. Used with permission.

W. H. Auden, 'The Model' and 'Musee des Beaux Arts' from *Collected Shorter Poems*
Reprinted by permission of Faber & Faber Ltd.

Simone de Beauvoir, from *A Very Easy Death,* translated by Patrick O'Brian (*Une Mort tres doure* published Librairie Gallimard, 1964, Great Britain by Andre Deutsch, Weidenfeld & Nicolson, 1966, Penguin Books 1969) © Librairie Gallimard, 1964. Translation © Andre Deutsch, Weidenfeld & Nicolson and G. P. Putnam's Sons, 1966. Reprinted by permission of Penguin Books Ltd.

Hilaire Belloc, from *Complete Verse* (Pimlico, a division of Random Century). Reprinted by permission of the Peters Fraser & Dunlop Group Ltd.

John Berger and Jean Mohr, from *A Fortunate Man* (Allen Lane, The Penguin Press, 1967), © John Berger and Jean Mohr, 1967. Reprinted by permission of the publisher and author.

John Betjeman, from *Collected Poems.* Reprinted by permission of John Murray (Publishers) Ltd.

Robert Bly, 'Counting Small-Boned Bodies' from *Selected Poems* (Harper & Row, New York), © Robert Bly, 1986. Used with permission.

George Mackay Brown, extract from 'The Shroud' from *Fisherman with Ploughs.* Reprinted by permission of John Murray (Publishers) Ltd.

Fanny Burney, from *The Journals and Letters of Fanny Burney,* vol. VI, ed. Joyce Hemlow, © OUP 1975. Reprinted by permission of Oxford University Press.

Anton Chekhov, 'Ward 6' from *Lady with Lapdog and Other Stories*, translated by David Magarshack (Penguin Classics, 1964), © David Magarshack, 1964. Reprinted by permission of Penguin Books Ltd.

Douglas Dunn, from *Elegies*. Reprinted by permission of Faber & Faber Ltd.

T. S. Eliot, extract from Act Two of *The Cocktail Party*; Section IV from 'Little Gidding' from *Four Quartets*. Reprinted by permission of Faber & Faber Ltd.

U. A. Fanthorpe, from *Selected Poems*.

Michael Flanders & Donald Swan, from *At the Drop of a Hat*.

E. M. Forster, from *Howard's End*. Reprinted by permission of King's College, Cambridge and The Society of Authors as the literary representatives of the E. M. Forster Estate.

Galen, 'A Case History' from *Source Book of Medical History*, ed. Logan Clendening (1960). Reprinted by permission of Dover Publications, Inc.

Janice Galloway, from *The Trick is to Keep Breathing* (Polygon/Minerva, n.e. 1994). © Janice Galloway.

Robert Graves, from *Collected Poems 1975*. © 1975 by Robert Graves. Reprinted by permission of Oxford University Press, Inc., and A. P. Watt Ltd on behalf of The Trustees of the Robert Graves Copyright Trust.

Thom Gunn, from *Jack Straw's Castle*. Reprinted by permission of Faber & Faber Ltd.

Seamus Heaney, 'Mid Term Break'. Reprinted by permission of Faber & Faber Ltd.

Joseph Heller, 'The Texan' from *Catch 22*, © 1955, 1961, 1989 by Joseph Heller. Reprinted by permission of Simon & Schuster, Inc., and A. M. Heath.

Hippocrates, from *Hippocratic Writings*, translated by J. Chadwick, W. N. Mann and edited by G. E. R. Lloyd (Penguin Classics, 1978), © J. Chadwick and W. N. Mann, 1950. Reprinted by permission of Penguin Books Ltd.

Terence Hirst, from *Apollo*. Reprinted by permission of the author.

Miroslav Holub, from *Vanishing Lung Syndrome*, translated by David Young and Dana Habova. Reprinted by permission of Faber & Faber Ltd.

B. Hurwitz and Ruth Richardson, 'Inspector General James Barry MD: putting the woman in her place', 'Jeremy Bentham's Self-Image', *British Medical Journal*, Vol. 298, 4 February 1989. 'The Life of Dr John Polidori', *Proceedings of the Royal College of Physicians, Edinburgh*. Reprinted by permission of the authors.

Elizabeth Jennings, from *Collected Poems* (Macmillan). Reprinted by permission of David Higham Associates Ltd.

Jenny Joseph, from *Selected Poems* published by Bloodaxe Books Ltd. © Jenny Joseph 1992 (US Distributors: Dufours). Reprinted by permission of John Johnson (Authors' Agent) Limited.

Dr Merrilees Karr, 'Mothers' from *The Moment of Death—A Comedy*, in *Journal of American Medical Association*, Nov. 4, 1988, Vol. 260, # 17. © Dr. Merrilees Karr 1988. Used with permission.

Jackie Kay, from *The Adoption Papers* (Bloodaxe Books, 1991), © Jackie Kay 1991.

James Kirkup, from *A Correct Compassion and Other Poems* (OUP). Reprinted by permission of the author.

Philip Larkin, 'This Be the Verse', 'Afternoons', 'The Old Fools', 'Ambulances', 'The Building',

'Ignorance', and 'Cut Grass' from *Collected Poems*. Reprinted by permission of Faber & Faber Ltd. 'At Grass' from *The Less Deceived*. Reprinted by permission of The Marvell Press.

D. H. Lawrence, 'Malade' from *The Complete Poems of D. H. Lawrence*, © 1964, 1971 by Angelo Ravagli and C. M. Weekley, Executors of the Estate of Frieda Lawrence Ravagli. Used by permission of Viking Penguin, a division of Penguin Books USA Inc.

C. S. Lewis, from *A Grief Observed*.

Penelope Lively, from *Passing On* (Penguin Books, 1990), © Penelope Lively, 1989. Reprinted by permission of Penguin Books Ltd.

Edward Lowbury, from *Selected and New Poems* (Hippopotamus Press, 1990). Reprinted by permission of the publisher and author.

Norman Maclean, from *A River Runs Through It* (1976). Reprinted by permission of the Estate of Norman F. Maclean and the University of Chicago Press.

Maimonides, from *The Guide of the Perplexed*, translated by Shlomo Pines (1963). Reprinted by permission of the University of Chicago Press.

Edna St. Vincent Millay, from *Collected Poems*, HarperCollins. Copyright 1923, 1951 by Edna St. Vincent Millay and Norma Millay Ellis. Reprinted by permission of Elizabeth Barnett, Literary Executor.

Michel de Montaigne, from *Essays*, translated by J. M. Cohen (Penguin Classics, 1958), © J. M. Cohen, 1958. Reprinted by permission of Penguin Books Ltd.

Edwin Muir, from *Collected Poems*. Reprinted by permission of Faber & Faber Ltd.

From *The Musician's World: Letters of the great composers*, edited by Hans Gal. © Thames & Hudson, London 1965. Used with permission.

Pablo Neruda, 'To the Foot from its Child', from *European Poetry in Scotland*, ed. Peter France and Duncan Glen (Edinburgh University Press). Used with permission.

Michael O'Donnell, 'Killjoy was here', *The Guardian*, 15 May 1985. Used with permission.

Wilfred Owen, 'Conscious' from *Poems of Wilfred Owen*. © 1963 by Chatto & Windus Ltd. Reprinted by permission of New Directions Publishing Corporation and Random House UK Ltd.

Paracelsus, from *Selected Writings*, ed. J. Jacobi, translated N. Guterman (1988). Reprinted by permission of Princeton University Press.

Dorothy Parker, from *Collected Dorothy Parker*. Reprinted by permission of Duckworth.

Samuel Pepys, excerpts from *Diary of Samuel Pepys: a new and complete transcription*, edited by Robert Latham and William Matthews, 11 volumes, © 1972–1986 The Master, Fellows and Scholars of Magdalene College, Cambridge, Robert Latham, and the Executors of William Matthews. Reprinted by permison of the University of California Press and Bell & Hyman, now Unwin Hyman, an imprint of Harper Collins Publishers Limited.

L. Peters, from *Satellites*. Reprinted by permission of Heinemann Publishers (Oxford) Ltd.

Robert M. Pirsig, from *Zen and the Art of Motorcycle Maintenance*, © Robert M. Pirsig 1974. Reprinted by permission of The Bodley Head and William Morrow, New York.

Sylvia Plath, 'Morning Song' from *Ariel*. Reprinted by permison of Faber & Faber Ltd.

Kathleen Raine, 'Spell of Sleep'. Reprinted by permission of the author.

Tessa Ransford, from *Fools and Angels* (1984). Reprinted by permission of The Ramsay Head Press.

Theodore Roethke, from *Collected Poems*. Reprinted by permission of Faber & Faber Ltd.

Oliver Sacks, from *The Man Who Mistook His Wife for a Hat* (Duckworth). © Oliver Sacks.

Fiona Sampson, from *Picasso's Men* (Phoenix Press), © Fiona Sampson 1993. Used with permission.

Seneca, from *Letters from a Stoic*, translated by Robin Campbell (Penguin Classics, 1969), © Robin Alexander Campbell, 1969. Reprinted by permission of Penguin Books Ltd.

Anne Sexton, from *All My Pretty Ones*. © 1962 by Anne Sexton, © renewed 1990 by Linda G. Sexton. Reprinted by permission of Houghton Mifflin Company and Sterling Lod Literistic Agency. All Rights Reserved.

Brian Sheldon, 'A Pharmaceutical Nightmare'. Reprinted by permission of the author.

Penelope Shuttle, from *The Orchard Upstairs* (OUP). Reprinted by permission of David Higham Associates Ltd.

Jon Silkin, from *Selected Poems*. Reprinted by permission of Routledge & Kegan Paul.

Stevie Smith, from *The Collected Poems of Stevie Smith* (Penguin 20th Century Classics). Reprinted by permission of James MacGibbon and New Directions Publishing Corporation.

Stephen Sondheim, 'Gee Officer Krupke' from *Westside Story*. © Stephen Sondheim.

Susan Sontag, from *Illness as a Metaphor* (Allen Lane, 1979), © Susan Sontag, 1977, 1978. Reprinted by permission of Penguin Books Ltd.

Jon Stallworthy, 'The Source'. © Jon Stallworthy.

Anne Stevenson, from *Selected Poems 1956–1986*, © Anne Stevenson, 1987. Reprinted by permission of Oxford University Press.

John Stone, from *In All This Rain*. © 1980 by John Stone. Reprinted by permission of Louisiana State University Press.

Dylan Thomas, from *The Poems*. Copyright 1945 by the Trustees for the copyrights of Dylan Thomas. Reprinted by permission of David Higham Associates Ltd. and New Directions Publishing Corp.

Alice Walker, from *Living by the Word* (The Women's Press). Reprinted by permission of David Higham Associates Ltd. (and Wendy Weil Agency).

Geoffrey Warnock, from *The Object of Morality* (Methuen, 1971). Used with permission.

Evelyn Waugh, from *Brideshead Revisited*, and *The Loved One*. Reprinted by permission of the Peters Fraser & Dunlop Group Ltd.

William Carlos Williams, from *Collected Poems 1909–1939, Volume I*. Copyright 1938 by New Directions Publishing Corp. Reprinted by permission of Carcanet Press Limited and New Directions. 'Le Medecin Malgre Lui' from *Doctor Stories*. Reprinted by permission of Faber & Faber Ltd.

John Wisdom, 'What is there in Horse-Racing?', *The Listener*, 10 June 1954. © 1954 *The Listener* and John Wisdom.

Ludwig Wittgenstein, from *Tractatus Logico Philosophicus*, translated D. F. Pears & B. F. McGuinness. Reprinted by permission of Routledge & Kegan Paul.

Any errors or omissions in the above list are entirely unintentional. If notified the publisher will make any necessary corrections at the earliest opportunity.

INDEX OF MEDICAL OR NURSING AUTHORS OR ⊰ ARTISTS ⊱

✠ INDEX OF AUTHORS ✠

INDEX OF FIRST LINES OF ❧ POEMS ❧